"Sean is a talented and knowledgeable fitness instructor that I am proud to have had the privilege of working with. Beyond his technical skill and knowledge, he also has a personality that makes him easy to get along with, and helps him inspire everyone, regardless of age, skill level, or gender, to become active through yoga and Pilates. This book is going to be a standard for athletes that are interested in taking their game to the next level in non-traditional fitness areas."

—Dean Pohlman, owner of Man Flow Yoga

"Sean teaches a challenging yet super fun yoga class. He is a master at what he does."

—Heather Kapande, owner of Nick's Pro Fitness

"Sean brings a lightness to any heavy-duty workout. His sense of humor keeps you smiling when your mind is telling you to frown and possibly give up. In my opinion, a light and kind teacher that can also encourage you to meet your edge is a treasure—and Sean is that!"

—Adriene Mishler of Yoga with Adriene

"Sean's power yoga workouts are my go-to yoga workouts. He is an amazing instructor and I love the way he always makes me laugh."

—Laura London of Laura London Fitness

"I was in search of inspiration for yoga and Pilates and when I found Sean online, I felt like I could accomplish my fitness goals and have fun at the same time! I had taken many different classes in person and online, but never did I connect with someone in such a human way. Sean is kind and thorough, yet silly enough to take your mind off of the many plankorific poses he teaches! His style of teaching is inclusive and full of variety, so you will never get bored. This combination makes for a long-term commitment from his students who keep coming back time and time again. I was so inspired by Sean that I became a yoga teacher myself!"

—Natalie Cummings, founder Cardio Yoga Fusion

"Working out with Sean is a blast! I refer my online clients to him because I know not only will they get a safe and effective workout, they are sure to be entertained in the process!"

—Dana Chapman of RealFitTV

"I love Sean's dedication to yoga and working out, his fun personality, and his commitment to helping people."

—Ali Kamenova of Ali Kamenova Yoga

"I love Sean's classes! He's my go-to power yoga instructor."

—Peggy Tung, owner of Core Solutions Pilates and Wellness

POWER YOGA

FOR ATHLETES

More than 100 Poses and Flows to Improve Performance in Any Sport

SEAN VIGUE

Fair Winds Press
100 Cummings Center, Suite 406L
Beverly, MA 01915

fairwindspress.com • bodymindbeautyhealth.com

© 2015 Fair Winds Press
Photography © 2015 Terri Zollinger

First published in the USA in 2015 by
Fair Winds Press, a member of
Quarto Publishing Group USA Inc.
100 Cummings Center
Suite 406-L
Beverly, MA 01915-6101
www.fairwindspress.com
Visit www.bodymindbeautyhealth.com. It's your personal guide to a happy, healthy, and extraordinary life!

19 18 17 16 15   1 2 3 4 5

ISBN: 978-1-59233-615-9
Digital edition published in 2015
eISBN: 978-1-62788-294-1

Library of Congress Cataloging-in-Publication Data
Vigue, Sean.
  Power yoga for athletes : more than 100 poses and flows to improve performance in any sport / Sean Vigue.
      pages cm
  ISBN 978-1-59233-615-9 (paperback)
  1. Astanga yoga 2. Athletes--Training of. I. Title.
  RA781.68.V54 2015
  613.7'046--dc23
                            2014049290
Cover design by Traffic
Book design by Traffic
Page layout by Sylvia McArdle
Photography by Terri Zollinger

Printed and bound in China

The information in this book is for educational purposes only. It is not intended to replace the advice of a physician or medical practitioner. Please see your health care provider before beginning any new health program.

Dedicated to my loving parents, Robert and Beverly, for their constant support, love, and encouragement. I love you!

CONTENTS

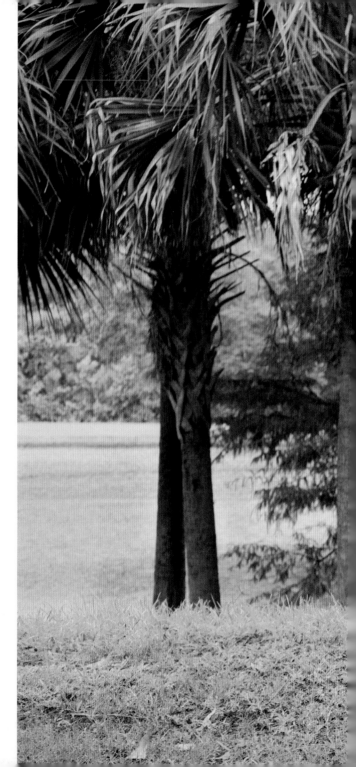

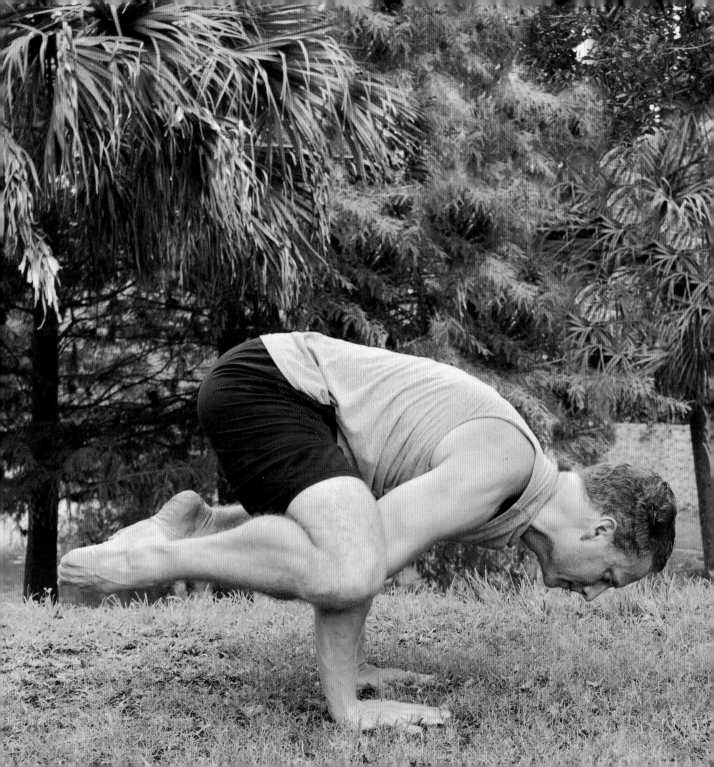

INTRODUCTION

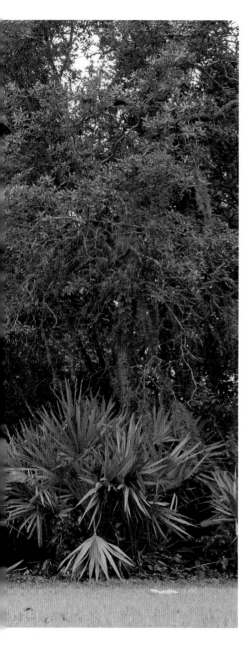

"Range is for the ego, control is for the soul."
—*Joseph Pilates*

Whatever your sport of choice, yoga can help you improve focus, flexibility, and performance. Power yoga in particular, a form of yoga involving aerobic exercises and constant strenuous movement, is ideal for athletes who strive for a holistic, balanced fitness routine and who want a strong, flexible body and better performance in the sport of their choice. Studies show that most athletes are used to conditioning in a particular way, usually by isolating specific muscle groups with the aim of increasing the intensity and frequency of the training regimen; this kind of conditioning focuses on isolating different parts of the body. Yoga, on the other hand, is based on the principle of integrating the body as a whole and shifts the emphasis to the quality of the movement. This holistic approach can reveal weaknesses and imbalances that may never have been exposed before. This may come as a surprise to many athletes who think they are in tune with their bodies.

This book, with more than one hundred power yoga poses plus yoga flows, is designed specifically for athletes who want a total body/mind workout. Yoga is the ideal cross-training tool and a perfect stand-alone exercise, whether you're looking to improve balance, focus, control, breathing, posture, or flexibility; strengthen your back, joints, or core; or reduce or heal from injury. Each yoga pose features step-by-step directions, instructional photography, and lists of the muscles being worked, the overall benefits, and the sports for which each pose is ideal. These poses benefit athletes of all types, including runners, swimmers, cyclists, golfers, and baseball, basketball, soccer, and American football players. When you incorporate these poses into a vigorous flow (chapters 9, 10, and 11), it becomes *power yoga*.

WHY DO POWER YOGA?

Power yoga is the athlete's secret weapon. Dozens of high-profile professional athletes are hitting the yoga mat, from the Seattle Seahawks American football team to basketball star LeBron James to the New Zealand All Blacks rugby team. Professional athletes are turning to power yoga to improve performance, prevent injury, and extend their careers. But while the word has gotten out that yoga is a natural fit for athletes, many are still too intimidated to give it a try. They view it as too "earthy," for "granolas," too intimidating, or foreign to their typical workout routine. But anyone who has practiced yoga could talk about its many benefits. Yoga involves movements and body postures that provide a full-body workout and improve flexibility, balance, focus, awareness, strength, endurance, and recovery. My hope is that *Power Yoga for Athletes* will serve as a gateway to all athletes interested in reaping the benefits the mat has to offer.

As a former professional singer/dancer and yoga instructor, I have seen firsthand the difference yoga can make to an athlete's performance. I also grew up playing hockey, football, basketball—you name it, I played it, and my goal is still to have that kind of unlimited energy throughout each day. Power yoga gives me that energy. In my life prior to becoming a yoga/Pilates instructor, grueling rehearsals and performances took their toll on my body. My muscles would feel tight, and my energy levels were dropping, affecting not only my rehearsals and performance but also my sleep. Plus, my focus wasn't as sharp as many of my fellow performers, and I had a hard time remembering all the complex music, lines, and choreography. I noticed that my fellow dancers who practiced yoga didn't seem to have the aches and

pains that I had. When I began practicing yoga, I noticed immediately how my body became stronger and my focus was as sharp as a laser. I was fortunate that a couple of fellow performers were yoga instructors, and they began to teach me some power yoga flows, which made my muscles long, lean, and powerful.

I began teaching yoga classes to small groups and eventually worked my way up to leading packed power yoga classes at the largest health club in the southwest United States. The combination of releasing the tensions of the day and building powerful, functional muscles while moving through sequences of poses, stretches, and meditations was equally appealing to desk jockeys as well as hardened athletes. In my experience as a yoga instructor, I see the incredible demand from athletes for a yoga experience that is tailored to their needs. And it makes sense. The benefits of power yoga for athletes abound.

Injury Prevention

Athletes repetitively overuse certain muscle groups, and most athletes are overdeveloped in certain areas and underdeveloped in others. This causes imbalances in strengthening and lengthening. These overdeveloped muscles become tight, pulling on ligaments and joints, decreasing the athlete's range of motion. For instance, runners tend to have tight hamstrings; cyclists often have tight quadriceps; those engaged in throwing sports or swimming may complain of tired or aching shoulders; golfers and tennis players may have more freedom of rotation in one direction than the other. More flexibility in the muscles can prevent injuries. Yoga is designed to

work the muscles around the joints for stability and full mobility.

Increased Performance

In addition to helping prevent injury, better flexibility and range of motion will add up to better performance. For example, LeBron James credits his amazing stamina to his yoga practice. "Yoga isn't just about the body, it's also about the mind, and it's a technique that has really helped me," James says. The full-body conditioning of yoga is the ultimate cross-training for all athletic endeavors.

Body Awareness

Proprioception is the ability to perceive the body with your mind. Yoga gives you a keener sense of how your body moves, which in turn helps with reaction time, as well as balance and injury prevention. It's your body, so you better know how to use it to its maximum potential!

Mind and Body Balance

Building better balance and coordination translates to better control over your body and how you use it. We've learned that yoga emphasizes working your mind and body as a whole instead of isolating certain areas of your body. As a result, your body moves more efficiently, and your form and technique improve. For instance, a tennis player may have more power in her forehand than backhand because of an imbalance in her body. By correcting this imbalance through yoga, her forehand and backhand become equally effective.

Core Strength

Core strength is one of the most important results of developing a yoga practice. A strong core (abdominals, lower back, hips, and gluteus) is extremely important to maintaining a healthy spine, because it can take pressure off the spine and help prevent injury. Being an athlete with a powerful core has many other benefits, including improved posture, better balance, less back pain, and easier breathing.

Breath Awareness

Yoga teaches us to become aware of our breath. This awareness allows us to strengthen the diaphragm and expand our lung tissue to its full capacity, which in turn increases the amount of oxygen that feeds the body and muscles, resulting in increased endurance.

Mental Focus

Yoga teaches us to be present in the moment. This allows us to block out the stimulus and noise that is always around us. Any athlete knows how important this focus is to performance.

Stress Relief

During performance and training, an athlete is constantly bombarded with stress and physical challenge. In contrast, yoga is called a moving meditation and teaches us how to calm the nervous system. Every athlete can put this skill into practice to quiet this stress and better attain mental focus.

Recovery Time

Studies have shown that athletes can come to a full recovery from injury through yoga practice. Indeed, yoga therapy is a growing method of physical therapy for injury recovery widely recognized by Western medicine. In addition, yoga helps with post-workout recovery time.

Endurance

All of the benefits above add up to an increase in stamina and endurance for competition. The athlete who lasts the longest usually wins the competition.

HOW TO USE THIS BOOK

My aim with *Power Yoga for Athletes* is to provide a guide that will get athletes on the mat with no fuss. The style of yoga incorporated in this book is commonly known as power yoga. Power yoga is simply a series of poses (asanas) that flow from one to the next with an emphasis on breath, strength, control, and flexibility. Power yoga brings yoga into the gym for people who want to work hard and build up a sweat. This is a guide that any athlete can pick up and begin using wherever they are. Each of the one hundred–plus diverse yoga poses will identify which muscles they target (see diagrams identifying body parts, front and back, on each page). You'll find the poses that are best for each sport by

finding the sport's icon at the bottom of each page—or in the training log found at the back of the book. Once you practice these poses, you can really get flowing with the 27 flows presented toward the end of the book.

Ready to get started? I've included eleven warm-up/cool-down flows that will stretch your entire body as well as calm your mind and ease you into the full workouts. Look for morning and evening routines, too. There are power flows, which are fourteen short but challenging routines for all fitness levels. Ready to really sweat? There are two massive endurance flows, which are complete power yoga workouts that will have your

heart pumping, your muscles glistening, and the sweat pouring as you train to become the best in your sport. The endurance flows are also available online via my YouTube channel (youtube.com/motleyfitness), so we can work out together, and you can see the flows in more detail. Also, look for a complete training log at the back of this book that will tell you the best poses for each sport. *Power Yoga for Athletes* is in essence a complete yoga training manual that you can take anywhere.

WHAT YOU NEED

I strongly recommend getting a thin yoga mat that you can roll up and take anywhere you wish to practice. Be careful that the mat isn't too thick and "squishy," or you'll have trouble holding steady because the mat will jiggle around. You may also practice on a soft surface such as grass, as I do in my videos, but you may have to deal with insects, dry patches of grass, and allergies. Use exercise straps or a small towel (also to wipe away all the sweat) to assist you in the Mudra poses if you're unable to bring your hands together. Keep a bottle of water handy to stay hydrated before, during, and after your workout. Wear your favorite workout clothes, and make sure they're loose fitting and comfortable; be ready to get sweaty.

WHEN TO PRACTICE

One of the best things about *Power Yoga for Athletes* is that it can fit into even the busiest of schedules. You can do it first thing in the morning, as a stand-alone workout, before or after your current workout, as a de-stressing workout, or right before you go to bed. This book contains flows for all these occasions, from warm-up and cool-down routines to full-blown power yoga sweat fests for an incredible total-body conditioning workout. Experiment, try different times, vary the workouts, and see what works best for you. You can also use these poses and flows for your recovery phases because they will keep your body refreshed, rejuvenated, and flexible. Your yoga journey is your own. Keep growing in your practice.

LISTEN TO YOUR BODY

It's always a good idea to consult your physician before beginning a yoga practice. Listen to your body. Be aware of how you feel and how the poses affect you. Yoga will always meet you exactly where you need it to if you just listen. There should never be pain in your yoga practice. If pain occurs, you may decide to stop or use one of the many modifications included in this book. It only takes a second to modify, and you can still keep the flow going. Take a quick breather and stay focused. Always be honest with yourself, be the master of your own practice, and make every power yoga workout an enjoyable and focused experience.

Are you ready to use this secret weapon? It's time you unleashed your full athletic potential and improve your performance on every level. Why give your rival the advantage when you have power yoga at your fingertips? This is your call to action. It's your time to be a champion. I'll meet you on the mat!

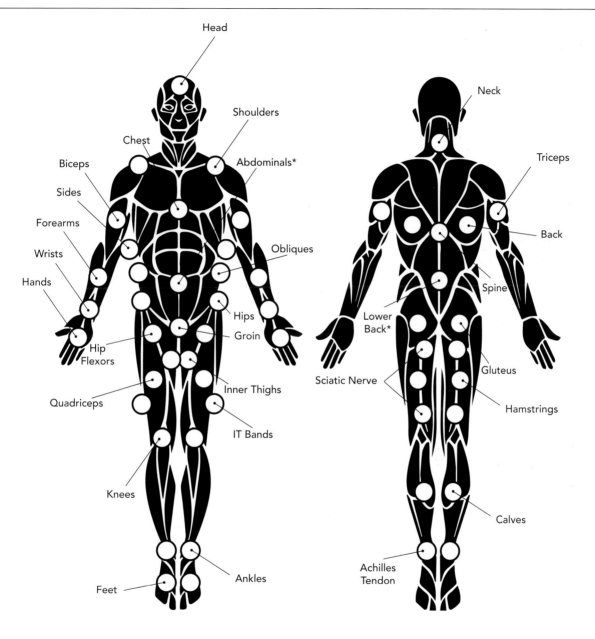

* Your abdominals and lower back make up your core.

ICONS EXPLAINED

 ### Running/Jogging

Runners are plagued by tight hamstrings, lower back, calves, hips, and shoulders, and that can slow you down. Every power yoga pose emphasizes stretching these crucial areas so you're not fighting against those tight muscles, but working in total harmony and constantly improving your stride and time.

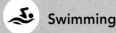 ### Swimming

Swimming can cause body misalignments, lack of bone strength and density, and very tight shoulders. Bones are living tissue and holding your weight up against gravity creates stress that increases your bone density. There are also plenty of poses to stretch tight shoulders and bring balance to your mind and body.

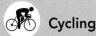 ### Cycling

Yoga is a wonderful partner for ripped legs, a strong heart, and tight hips. By keeping your muscles stretched and balanced, you'll be able to ride in the saddle for longer periods of time and have increased energy. The mind/body yoga connection will sharpen your focus for those long, grueling rides.

 ### Golf

I recently introduced my father to yoga because he was having flexibility issues with twisting, not to mention his backswing was suffering from decreased balance. He has experienced dramatic improvements in his core strength, control of the ball, and in his backswing power. He's now 80 years old and playing better than he has in years.

 ### Tennis

I played tennis for many years and always had problems balancing out my forearm and backhand—my weak backhand always suffered because of my lack of flexibility and core strength. Enter power yoga and my backhand became extra powerful and deadly accurate, not to mention my endurance and focus began to blow away the competition.

 ### Baseball/Cricket

In baseball you have to keep your body always at the ready even as you are forced to sit or stand for long periods of time. Power yoga prepares your body for any athletic challenge by keeping all your muscles in a constant state of readiness and control. The focus on core strength and flexibility training will help you swing, run, and dive with greater ease and precision even when you're moving from a stationary position.

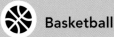 ### Basketball

Basketball is a tremendous workout requiring endurance, agility, and bursts of speed that can wear down and fatigue your body. Many top professional players have started utilizing yoga to stay flexible, build their ankle muscles, and give them added endurance to keep them running up and down the court smoothly.

 ### Hockey

It's no secret that hockey is my favorite sport and I had the pleasure of playing for about 10 years while growing up. It's also no secret that yoga poses will loosen and stretch your entire body while keeping your core, legs, gluteus, and hips strong and resistant to injury. Skate circles around your opponents and avoid career ending hits with regular practice of the poses in this book.

 ### American Football/ Rugby

You know who does yoga? The Super Bowl Champion Seattle Seahawks. More and more gridiron warriors are flocking to yoga classes to improve their functional strength, balance, flexibility, power, breathing efficiency, speed, and focus, not to mention making them more resistant to injury and providing longevity in one of the most physically brutal sports in history.

Soccer/Football

I played soccer for a few years and I swear it's the toughest cardio sport. The field is huge and you are in constant movement to get near the ball and slam it into the opponent's goal. The tremendous agility and endurance required on the field will be given a huge boost by adding yoga into your training and your risk of injury will decrease.

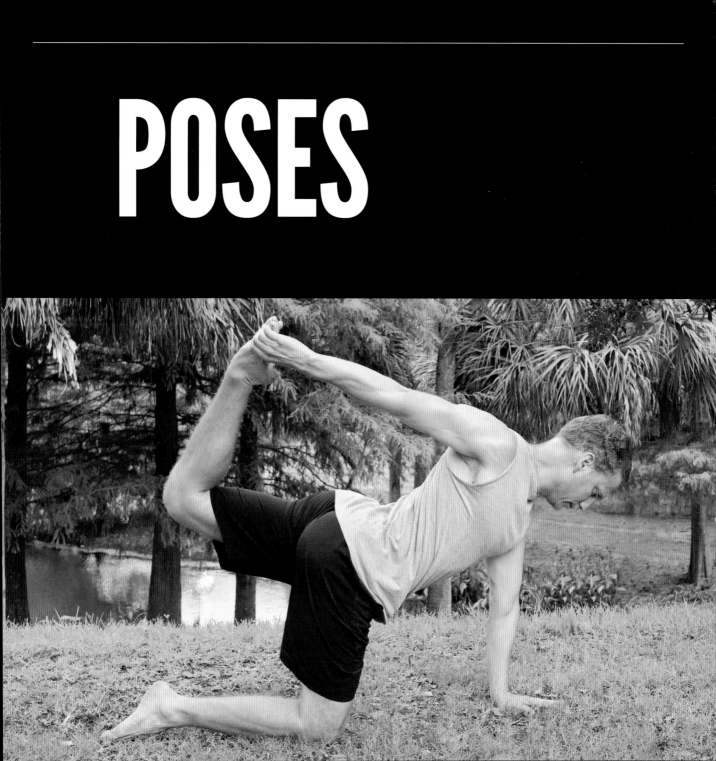

POSES

CHAPTER 1
WARM-UP AND FOCUS

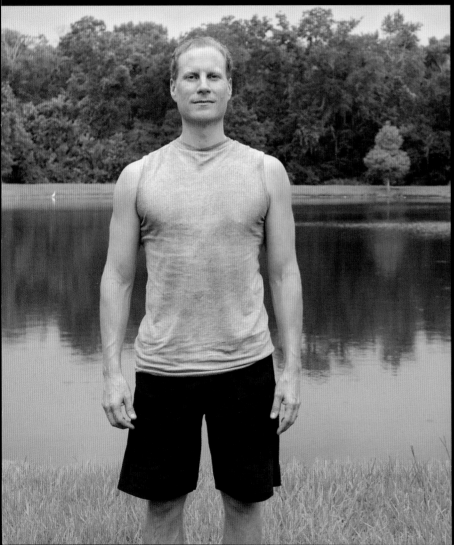

Your journey to a stronger, fitter, and more flexible body begins here. In these essential warm-up poses you'll find the door to escape into your power yoga workout. An effective warm-up can increase the blood flow to the working muscles, which results in decreased muscle stiffness, reduced risk of injury, and improved physical and mental performance. Every pose in this book begins with a breath, so make sure you're always breathing into your deep abdominals to drown your muscles in oxygen. To make sure your breath is going to the right spot, place your fingers around your belly button, and breathe in and out of your nostrils for five seconds. If your stomach "pooches" out, you're in the right spot! Spread that breath into your sides and lower back too for maximum oxygen uptake. Keep breathing in a steady rhythm. The deeper you breathe, the more energy, focus, and strength you will have. When learning these poses, I recommend holding each for five to ten deep breaths or thirty to sixty seconds for maximum mind/body connection. Ready to get started? Let's go!

MOUNTAIN

(Tadasana)

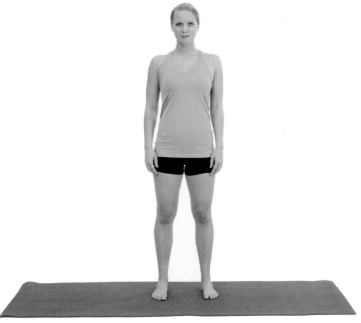

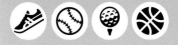

Stand tall! This is the pose to bring your mind, body, and spirit into your power yoga practice by adjusting your posture, tuning out the world, and turning your attention to your breath.

1. Stand with your feet hip-width apart and your arms at your sides.

2. Roll your shoulders back and down to create space between your ears and shoulders while tucking your chin slightly. Imagine gently holding an orange between your chin and your chest to open up the back of your neck and relax your jaw.

3. Breathe deep into your abdominal muscles for five to ten deep breaths, and give them a little squeeze as you exhale to get them fired up for what's to come.

Target body areas:

feet, ankles, quadriceps, hamstrings, and core.

Sports it benefits

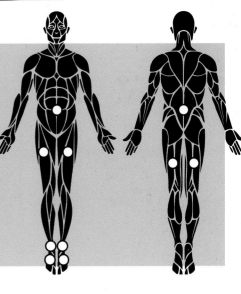

SIDE BEND
(Urdhva Hastasana)

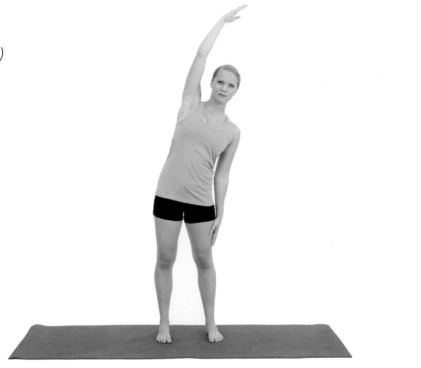

Stretch your sides, strengthen your thighs, and loosen up your spine with Side Bend.

1. From Mountain, inhale and extend your right arm, and exhale as you bend to the left.

2. Keeping your shoulders down and back, inhale and return to the center as you drop your right arm and extend your left.

3. Exhale and extend your left arm as you sway to the left.

Repeat five times on each side with deep breathing.

Target body areas:

feet, ankles, quadriceps, obliques, sides, and spine.

Sports it benefits

BACK BEND

(Anuvittasana)

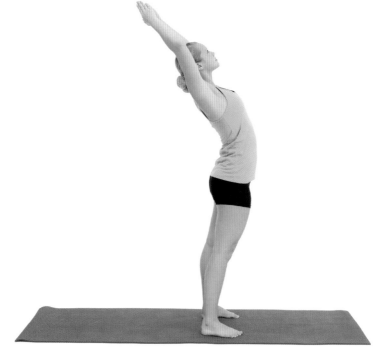

Here's a great pose to relieve stress in your lower back and open up your abdominals.

1. From Mountain, inhale and extend both arms up, while bringing your fingertips together.

2. As you exhale, gently bend backward, while keeping your shoulders relaxed and your thighs engaged.

3. Inhale and return to the standing position. Repeat five times, while taking deep breaths. You may hold the pose longer if desired.

Modification: Place your hands on your lower back for more support.

Target body areas:

feet, ankles, quadriceps, core, and chest.

Sports it benefits

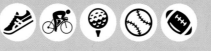

FORWARD FOLD
(Padangusthasana)

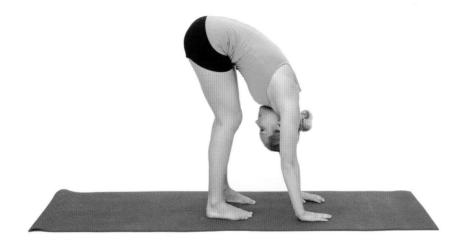

This is an amazing pose to unlock, open up, and de-stress your body.

1. From Mountain, inhale and bring your arms overhead, and exhale, while bending forward from your hips and unraveling your spine slowly toward the floor.

2. Keep your knees soft as you take deep breaths, and place your weight into your toes for maximum stretch.

3. Let your arms hang freely, while keeping your head and neck relaxed. Take five to ten deep breaths, and flex your abdominals with each exhale to protect and support your lower back.

4. Inhale and slowly return to standing by keeping your abdominals engaged and stacking your spine one vertebrae at a time. Repeat five times.

Target body areas:

calves, hamstrings, lower back, spine, neck, and head.

Sports it benefits

FLAT BACK

(Urdha Mulcha Uttanasana)

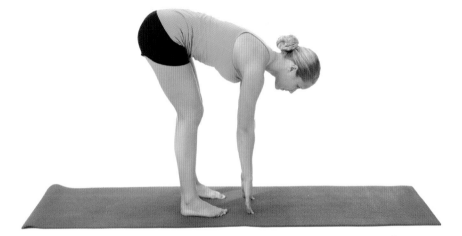

Need to really lengthen your spine? Let's do Flat Back!

1. From Forward Fold, inhale and place your fingertips on your shins or the floor, while keeping your shoulders back and your neck long.

2. Place your weight into your heels and lengthen your legs, while keeping your core tight, and take five to ten deep breaths. Release back to Forward Fold and repeat.

Modification: Place your fingertips on your shins.

Target body areas:

calves, hamstrings, core, spine, and shoulders.

Sports it benefits

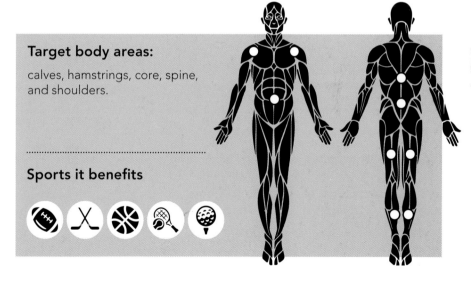

CHAPTER 2
FOUNDATION

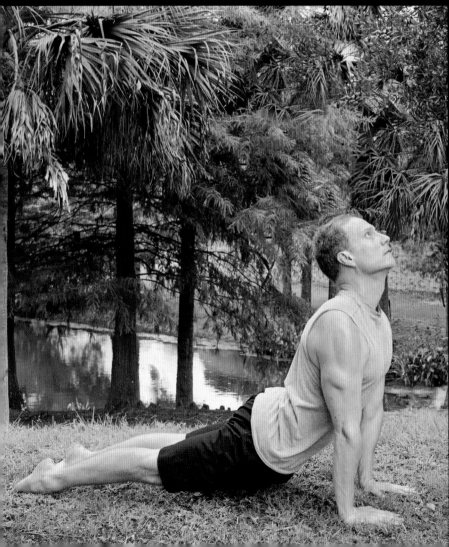

Athletes need strong physical and mental foundations in their training, and these are the classic poses to build that strong foun-dation. Developing the muscle memory of proper alignment in these poses will carry over into more challenging poses and result in a safer and stronger practice. Use this chapter to focus inward and begin treating your mind and body as equal partners in your fitness. I always strive to relearn and discover each pose for the first time when I practice. Even the most advanced yogis and athletes should never stop practicing the foundation poses of yoga. From these poses, your yoga practice shall arise.

Downward Facing Dog
(Adho Mukha Svanasana)

This pose is the absolute nucleus of power yoga because of all the poses that flow directly from it. Downward Facing Dog is a powerful stand-alone pose or the center of an exciting yoga flow. This intense stretch helps oxygen-rich blood flow to the head. Everyone should be doing Down Dog daily to improve their performance.

1. Begin in Forward Fold, and walk your hands forward until you've created a pyramid shape with your body.

2. Open your fingers wide, and relax your neck as you inhale and lift your tailbone toward the sky.

3. Exhale and sink your heels into the floor, lengthen your legs, and move your chest toward your legs. Hold for five to ten deep breaths.

Target body areas:

Achilles tendon, calves, hamstrings, spine, shoulders, neck, and head.

Sports it benefits

THREE LEGGED DOG
(Tri Pada Adho Mukha Svanasana)

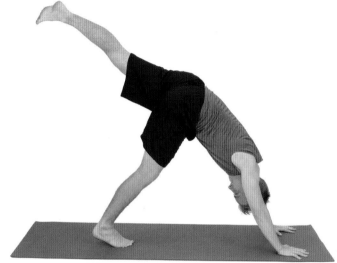

Build more balance, and take your Down Dog to the next level.

1. From Downward Facing Dog, inhale and lift your left leg toward the sky, while keeping your arms and core engaged to hold the balance.

2. With each inhale, lift your leg higher, and with each exhale, extend your arms more. Hold for five to ten deep breaths before repeating on the other side.

Target body areas:

Achilles tendon, calves, hamstrings, gluteus, hip flexors, core, triceps, and shoulders.

Sports it benefits

24

UPWARD FACING DOG

(Urdhva Mukha Svanasana)

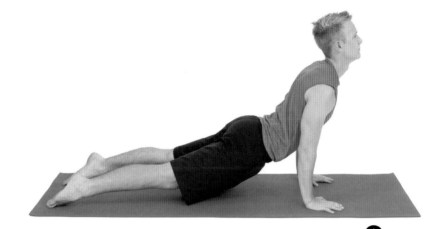

A great lower back and stomach stretch, and a nervous system stimulant—all in one.

1. From Downward Facing Dog, shift your weight forward to Plank (page 87), and slowly lower all the way to the floor.

2. Place your hands under your shoulders, adjust your feet so the tops of your feet are flat on the mat, inhale, and press your chest skyward, while keeping your gluteus and thighs engaged.

3. Roll your shoulders back and down to open your chest, and lift everything off the mat except your hands and the tops of your feet. Hold for five to ten deep breaths.

Modification: Drop your knees to the mat.

Target body areas:

core, chest, wrists, biceps, triceps, back, and shoulders.

Sports it benefits

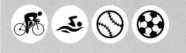

WIDE LEGGED DOWN DOG

(Adho Mukha Svanasana)

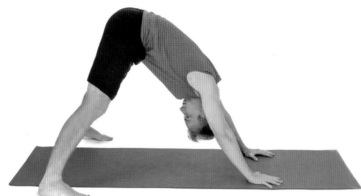

Achieve a massive spinal stretch from this Down Dog variation. This pose brings lots of oxygen to the brain.

1. From Down Dog, walk your feet to the outside edges of your mat.

2. Allow your chest to move farther toward your legs with each exhale.

3. Slowly sway your upper body side to side with each exhale, returning to the center as you inhale. Keep your heels down, and relax your head and neck. Hold for five to ten deep breaths.

Target body areas:

Achilles tendon, calves, hamstrings, inner thighs, spine, shoulders, and neck.

Sports it benefits

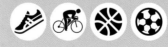

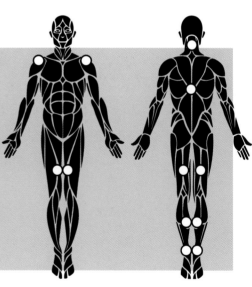

CHAIR
(Utkatasana)

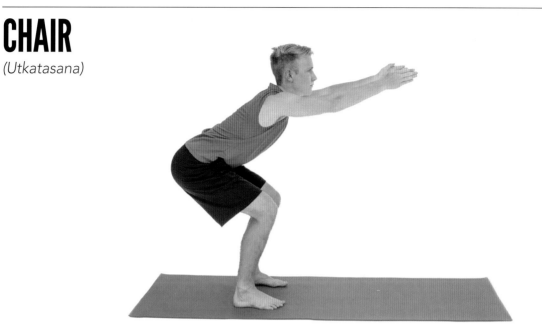

Need some energy? This pose will energize your whole body and build strong glutes and legs. It will also improve balance and focus.

1. From Mountain pose, exhale and press your bum back into a squat position by placing your weight into your heels and gluteus.

2. Inhale and reach your arms and chest to the sky, while keeping your shoulders relaxed. Spread your toes, and relax your fingers.

3. Press your bum back farther as you exhale, and lift your arms higher as you inhale. Your toes should be able to move freely. Hold for five to ten deep breaths.

Modification: Place your hands together in front of your heart (prayer position).

Target body areas:

ankles, Achilles tendon, calves, quadriceps, inner thighs, hips, gluteus, and lower back.

Sports it benefits

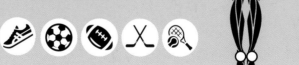

CAMEL
(Ustrasana)

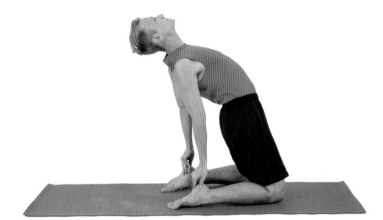

Camel really opens up the front of your body with an intense stretch that helps improve posture by correcting rounded shoulders. Camel also stimulates the kidneys and opens the breathing airways. *Skip this pose if you have lower back problems.*

1. Kneeling on your mat, place your knees hip-width apart, your hands on your lower back, and the tops of your feet on the mat.

2. Inhale as you lift taller, and press your hips forward. Slide your hands down to your heels as you continue to open your chest, while keeping your chin slightly tucked.

3. Exhale as you continue to press your hips, thighs, and stomach forward. Hold for five to ten deep breaths. Come out of the pose by returning to a kneeling position.

Modification: Keep your hands on your lower back.

Target body areas:

quadriceps, hip flexors, core, chest, and shoulders.

Sports it benefits

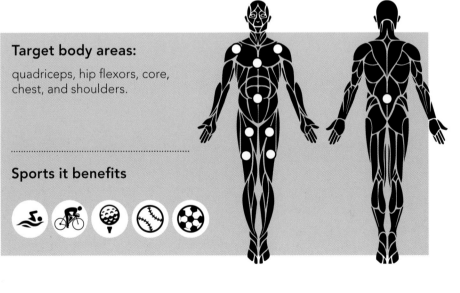

TALL MOUNTAIN
(Tadasana)

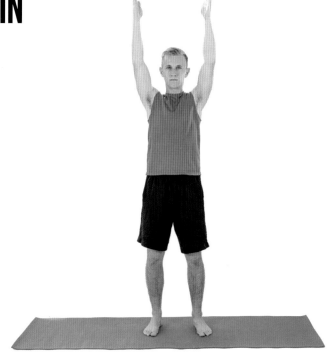

Stand tall and proud in this deeply rooted pose that improves posture and builds confidence and focus.

1. From Mountain pose, raise your arms overhead with your palms facing inward, while relaxing your shoulders down.

2. Feel your feet rooted in the earth and your fingertips reaching to the sky. Hold for five to ten deep breaths, and visualize the strength in your body.

Target body areas:

feet, ankles, quadriceps, core, and shoulders.

Sports it benefits

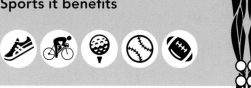

SHOULDER STAND
(Sarvangavana)

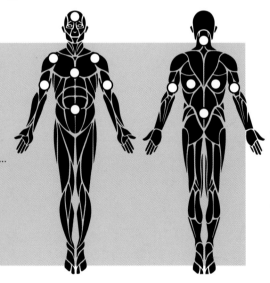

This just might be the most beloved of all the yoga poses. This pose builds balance and core strength, while increasing circulation to the thyroid glands and brain. It also calms and focuses the mind and body.

1. Lie on your back, and exhale as you lift your legs skyward. Place your hands on your lower back for support, and keep your eyes on your toes.

2. Straighten your legs in the air, extend your thighs, and point your toes.

3. Keep your chin tucked slightly and your neck relaxed as you bring your elbows closer together. Find the balance in your shoulders and core. Hold for five to ten deep breaths or until the pose is no longer comfortable, and then slowly lower your back down and bring your knees into your chest.

Modification: Keep your knees bent.

Target body areas:

core, chest, biceps, triceps, back, shoulders, neck, and head.

Sports it benefits

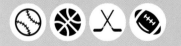

PLOW
(Halasana)

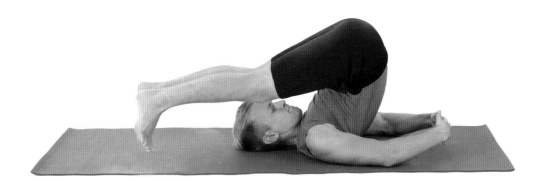

It's time to stimulate and rejuvenate your entire nervous system. This pose will also release tension in the neck and shoulders. Skip this pose if you have neck problems.

1. From Shoulder Stand, slowly extend your legs as you lower your feet over your head.

2. Keep your head and neck relaxed and your hands on your lower back for support. Try to touch your toes to the floor. Don't worry if you can't yet, but keep breathing into the stretch.

3. Keep your eyes upward, drop your arms to the floor, and lace your fingers together if you're able. Keep lengthening the legs slowly with each exhale, and relax your shoulders into the mat. Slowly bring your knees into your chest when you're done. Hold for five to ten deep breaths or until you're no longer comfortable.

Modification: Keep your knees bent, or keep your hands on your lower back.

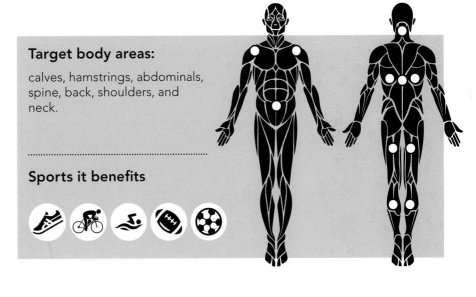

Target body areas:

calves, hamstrings, abdominals, spine, back, shoulders, and neck.

Sports it benefits

GATE
(Parighasana)

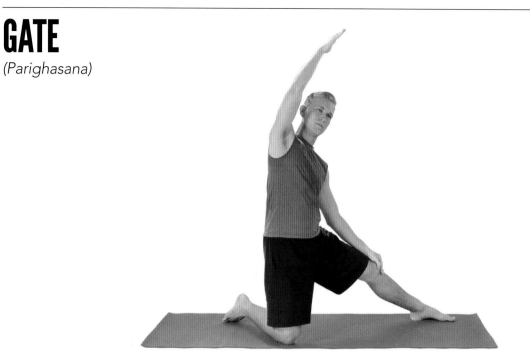

Open the gateway to more energy and super-stretched muscles along the spine.

1. Begin by kneeling on your mat with your knees hip-width apart, and extend your left foot to the left side, keeping your leg and foot in line with your hip.

2. Place your left hand on your left leg, inhale and extend your right arm overhead.

3. Exhale and bring your right arm into a side bend to the left, while sliding your left hand down your left leg. Keep your shoulders back and down, while pulling in your abs. Hold for five to ten deep breaths, return to the center on the inhale, and repeat on the other side.

Target body areas:

calves, hamstrings, inner thighs, sides, chest, and shoulders.

Sports it benefits

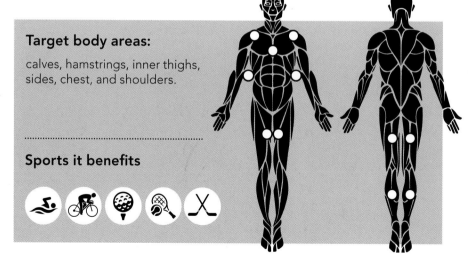

BOW
(Dhanurasana)

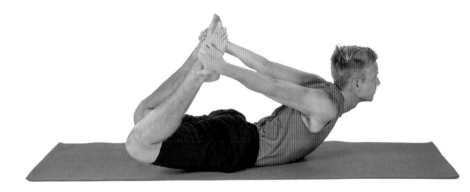

If you want a happy spine and loose quadriceps, drop down and do a Bow.

1. Lie on your stomach, and reach your arms to your sides, while bending your knees 90 degrees.

2. Lift your chest, press your pubic bone into the mat, and grab your feet or ankles. You may use a small towel or a strap if you're unable to reach your feet or ankles.

3. Press your toes to the sky, while lifting your chest and keeping your chin slightly tucked. Stretch your arms as much as possible, and pull your shoulders back. Hold for five to ten deep breaths or until it's not comfortable, and release.

Target body areas:

quadriceps, abdominals, chest, forearms, spine, and shoulders.

Sports it benefits

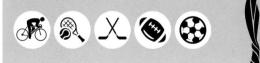

DOLPHIN
(Makarsana)

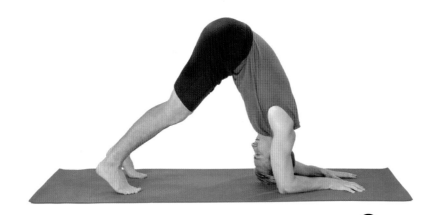

If you're looking for a yoga pose that builds strong arms and shoulders, Dolphin is a great choice.

1. From Downward Facing Dog, place your forearms on the floor, and walk your feet forward a few inches.

2. Exhale and move your chest toward your legs, while working your heels downward.

3. Keep your head and neck relaxed as you lift your tailbone upward. Hold for five to ten deep breaths, and bring your knees down.

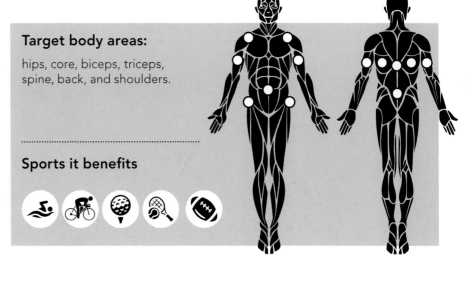

Target body areas:

hips, core, biceps, triceps, spine, back, and shoulders.

Sports it benefits

CROW
(Kakasana)

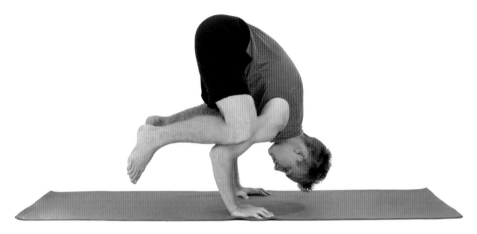

This powerful arm balance pose will build formidable upper body strength and balance.

1. Start in a crouching position with your hips open and your feet hip-width apart.

2. Place your hands on the floor with your arms on the inside of your thighs, and press your weight forward until your feet lift off the mat. Balance in Crow for five to ten deep breaths, and slowly release back down.

Modification: This is a very challenging pose, so start by rocking your weight forward and keeping your toes on the mat before progressing to a full lift off.

Target body areas:

core, wrists, forearms, biceps, triceps, and back.

Sports it benefits

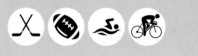

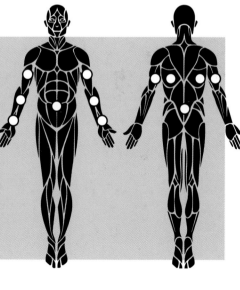

PIGEON

(Adho Mukha Eda Pada Rajakapotasana)

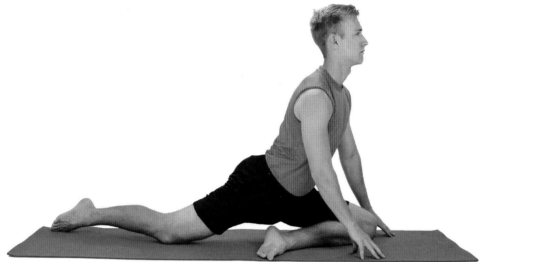

Tight hips lead to a really tight lower back. Luckily, Pigeon will revive both.

1. Begin in Down Dog, and bend and slide your left knee forward onto the mat, while extending your right leg behind you.

2. Open your left hip, and center your weight over the center of your body, while keeping your hands on the mat for support.

3. With each exhale, walk your hands farther forward, while opening your left hip and stretching your right hip flexor. Hold for five to ten deep breaths, and repeat with your right knee forward.

Target body areas:

hip flexors, groin, hips, gluteus, lower back, and spine.

Sports it benefits

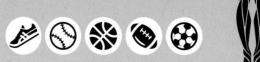

TIGER

(Vyaghrasana)

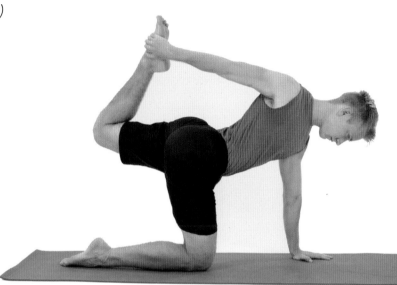

Loosen up and build balance as you become a Tiger. This pose relieves stress on the sciatic nerve, strengthens the core, and stretches the quadriceps.

1. Start in hands and knees position with your hands under your shoulders and your knees under your hips.

2. Extend your left leg behind you, and bend it 90 degrees, while reaching your right hand to your right side.

3. Grab your left foot with your right hand, and extend the toes upward, while keeping your knees centered. Hold for five to ten deep breaths. Release and repeat on other side.

Modification: Keep your right arm to your side, and hold the pose.

Target body areas:

quadriceps, hip flexors, core, spine, and shoulders.

Sports it benefits

CHAPTER 3
BALANCE

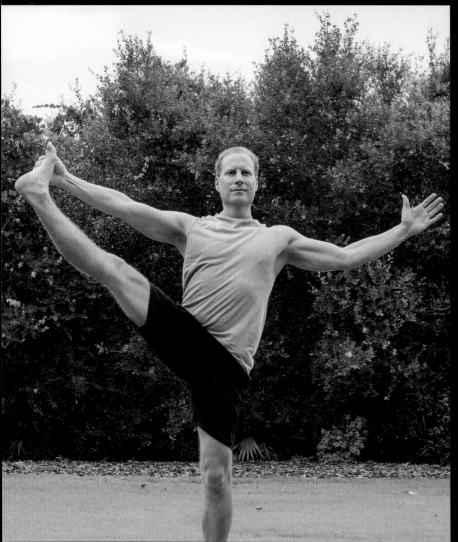

To be an elite athlete, you must have balance—balance of the mind, body, and spirit. Yoga balance poses are so powerful because they combine all three together in one unbreakable unit, in which one cannot exist without the other. Your whole being must work together to keep a balance pose stable. If you fall, no big deal—get right back up and try again. Their purpose is to teach us how to focus and persevere with integrity and humility. Balance poses also help us improve coordination, increase strength, and develop stability, while reducing stress and relieving fatigue. Let's find that focus that will keep you strong in any athletic endeavor.

TREE

(Vrksasana)

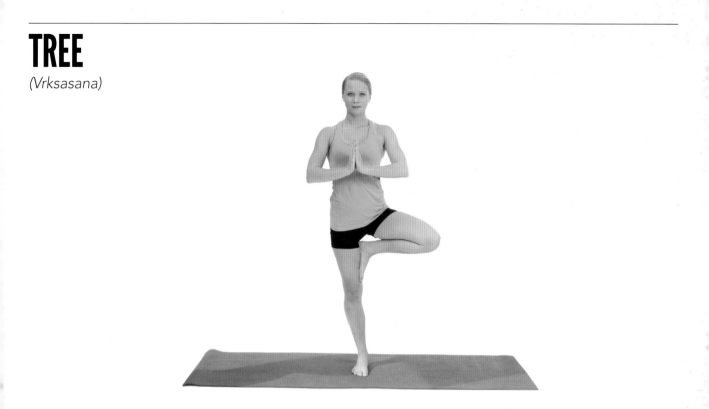

Learn to balance and focus in the roughest storm. This pose builds a stronger mind/body connection and focus, while improving posture.

1. From Mountain pose, put your hands together in front of your chest, while opening your left hip. Keep your shoulders relaxed.

2. Position your left foot below or above your knee on the inside of your right leg, and keep your right knee a little soft. As you exhale, give your abs a little squeeze.

3. Find a spot to focus on, and take five to ten deep breaths. Repeat on the other side.

Target body areas:

feet, ankles, calves, quadriceps, and core.

Sports it benefits

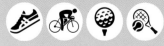

EXTENDED TREE

(Vrksasana)

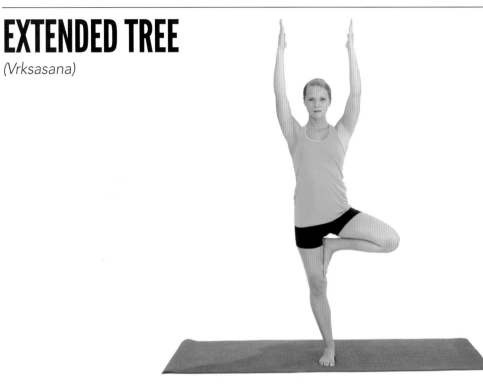

Take your Tree pose to the next level, offering even more balance and core engagement.

1. From Tree pose, extend your arms overhead with your palms facing inward.

2. Keep your shoulders relaxed, while taking five to ten deep breaths. Repeat on both sides.

Target body areas:

feet, ankles, calves, quadriceps, core, and shoulders.

Sports it benefits

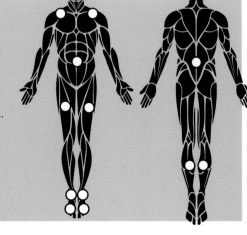

WILLOW

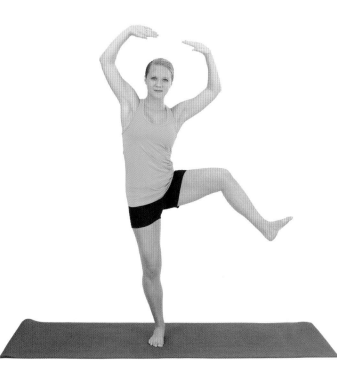

Take your Tree pose to an entirely different level as you open your hip and lift your entire body. This one works the gluteus and core even more.

1. From Tree pose, lift your left leg, and place it out to the side, while extending your arms and pressing your palms to the left and keeping your elbows bent.

2. Keep your left hip open, and flex your left foot, while continuing to press your palms to the left. Don't let your left leg sink. Hold for five to ten deep breaths, and repeat with your left foot on the floor.

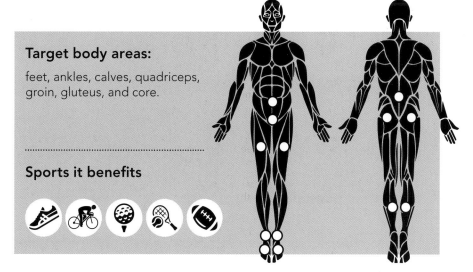

Target body areas:

feet, ankles, calves, quadriceps, groin, gluteus, and core.

Sports it benefits

HEAD TO KNEE

(Dandayamana Janushirasana)

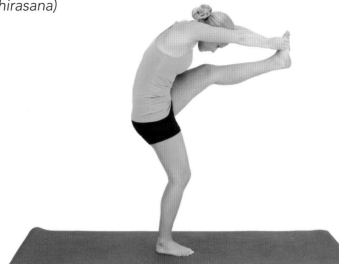

Burn some serious calories with this challenging Balance pose. It's fantastic for building focus, concentration, and balance.

1. Begin in a standing position, lace your fingers around your left hamstring, and draw your left knee into your chest.

2. Lace your fingers around the bottom of your left foot, and slowly extend your leg forward with an exhale. Lengthen your leg with each exhale, and draw your face toward your knee.

3. Straighten your arms as much as possible, while holding the pose for five to ten deep breaths. Repeat with your left foot on the floor.

Modification: Stop and hold when you draw your knee into your chest.

Target body areas:

feet, ankles, calves, sciatic nerve, hamstrings, quadriceps, biceps, and lower back.

Sports it benefits

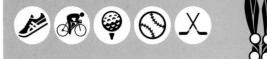

DANCER
(Natarajasana)

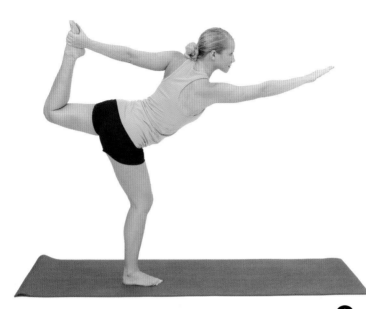

This graceful pose works your legs and upper arms and adds fire to your determination. It also opens the chest and lungs for better breathing. It's a great pose to develop greater balance, focus, and presence.

1. Begin in a standing position, extend your right arm forward, and grab the inside of your left foot behind you.

2. As you inhale, lift your left foot up, while extending your right arm forward and keeping your left knee in toward the center so your hips are square.

3. Stretch your left arm as much as possible, while keeping your chest lifted and your left foot lifting with each exhale. Hold for five to ten deep breaths, and keep your right knee slightly soft. Repeat with your left foot on the floor.

Target body areas:

feet, ankles, calves, quadriceps, core, spine, and shoulders.

Sports it benefits

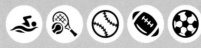

HALF RUSSIAN

(Utthita Hasta Padangusthasana B)

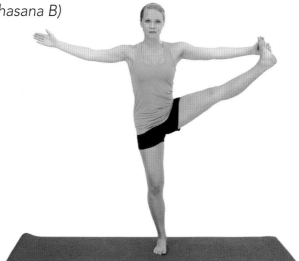

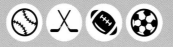

When you can't do the full, you must settle for the challenging Half Russian. This is a very challenging pose that requires a lot of core strength and control.

1. Begin in standing position, open your left hip, and grab your left ankle or foot with your left hand.

2. Extend your right arm to the right side for balance, while extending your left leg out to the side.

3. Keep your shoulders relaxed, your right knee soft, and extend your left arm fully. Hold for five to ten deep breaths, and repeat on the other side.

Modification: Grab your left hamstring with your left hand, and extend the left leg to the left, keeping your knee bent.

Target body areas:

feet, ankles, calves, quadriceps, inner thighs, hamstrings, groin, core, chest, and shoulders.

Sports it benefits

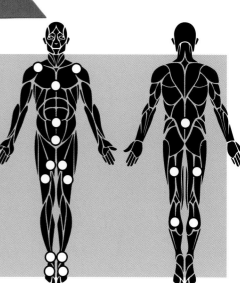

STANDING TWIST

(Parivrtta Hasta Padangusthasana)

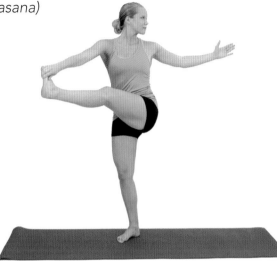

This pose creates a whole new twist on a standing balance pose, stretches your IT bands, and opens your breathing. It also improves balance and focus.

1. From a standing position, draw your left knee into your chest with your left hand.

2. Extend your left leg forward, and grab the outside of the ankle with your right hand.

3. Extend your left arm to the left as you draw your left leg to the right creating a twist. Turn your upper body to the left to fulfill the whole twist. Hold for five to ten deep breaths if you can stand it! Repeat with your left foot on the floor.

Modification: Keep your left knee bent, and grab the outside of the thigh with your right hand.

Target body areas:

ankles, calves, IT bands, quadriceps, hamstrings, hips, gluteus, and shoulders.

Sports it benefits

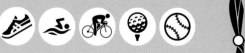

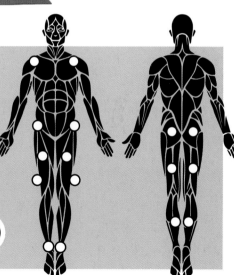

45

EAGLE

(Garudasana)

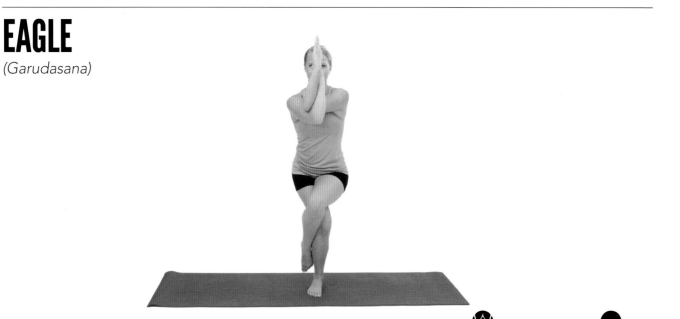

Soar high with my favorite yoga pose for opening the shoulders and building strength in your legs. This pose encourages extreme focus and confidence.

1. Press back into Chair pose, and extend your left arm forward, while wrapping your right arm underneath and around your left arm. Bring your palms together.

2. Wrap your left leg over your right, and keep your hips square to the front. Press your bum back farther.

3. Lift your fingers, relax your shoulders, and draw your elbows forward to really activate the pose. Find your focus, and hold for five to ten deep breaths. Repeat with your left leg on the floor and your left arm wrapping under your right.

Modification: Keep your lower body in a chair instead of wrapping your legs.

Target body areas:

feet, ankles, calves, quadriceps, core, wrists, forearms, back, and shoulders.

Sports it benefits

ONE-LEGGED CHAIR

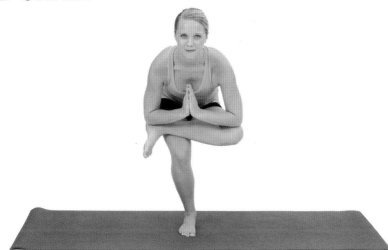

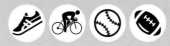

This is a fantastic leg, gluteus, and core workout in one. It brings together balance and focus and opens the hips.

1. Begin standing, and bring your hands together as you place your left ankle on your right thigh.

2. Press back into One-Legged Chair, placing the emphasis in your gluteus and right heel, while bringing your hands together in front of your chest.

3. Place your elbows on your left leg, and keep pressing into your gluteus muscles. Engage your core, and keep your upper body lifted. Hold for five to ten breaths, and repeat with your left foot on the floor.

Target body areas:

feet, ankles, calves, hamstrings, quadriceps, hips, gluteus, and core.

Sports it benefits

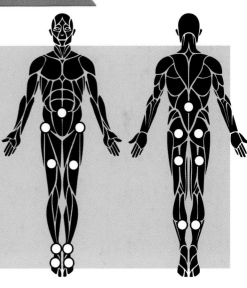

STAR

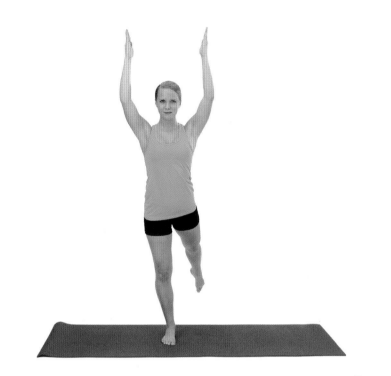

Be a bright, balanced star with this simple yet challenging pose. This one encourages better posture.

1. Begin in standing position, and draw your left leg back on a slight diagonal, while lifting your arms overhead.

2. Squeeze your gluteus, while lifting your leg back farther and relaxing your shoulders.

3. Soften your right knee slightly, and draw your arms back as far as possible. Hold for five to ten deep breaths, and repeat with your left foot on the floor.

Target body areas:

feet, ankles, calves, hamstrings, quadriceps, gluteus, lower back, and shoulders.

Sports it benefits

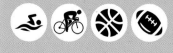

SHOOTING STAR

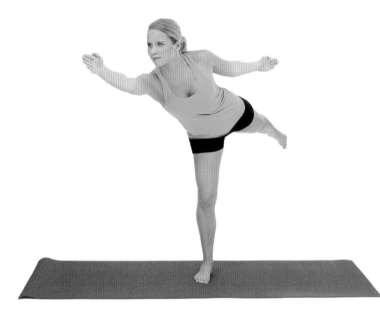

Lengthen your body, and challenge your focus. This pose improves balance and stability.

1. From Star pose, extend your left leg back farther, and reach your right arm farther forward.

2. Place your left arm in line with your left leg, and form a diagonal line, keeping your left hip slightly open. Hold for five to ten deep breaths, and repeat with your left foot on the floor.

Target body areas:

feet, ankles, calves, hamstrings, quadriceps, hips, gluteus, lower back, and shoulders.

Sports it benefits

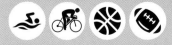

HALF MOON BALANCE

(Ardha Chandrasana)

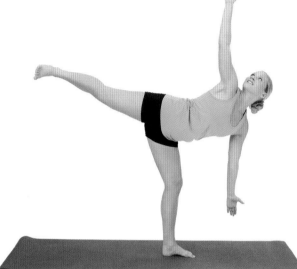

This pose improves your sense of balance and coordination. It's a perfect combination of balance, strength, and release—this pose has it all.

1. Stand with your feet about 3 feet (0.9 m) apart, and open your left hip. Your left toes should be pointing to your left.

2. Place your left hand on the floor about 1 foot (0.3 m) to the left of your left foot, and lift your right leg off the floor.

3. Extend your right arm upward as you open your right hip.

4. For the extreme balance, lift your left hand 1 inch (2.5 cm) off the floor, and look to your right hand. Flex your right foot, and keep lifting upward. Isn't this fun? Hold for five to ten deep breaths, and repeat with your right foot on the floor.

Target body areas:

feet, ankles, calves, hamstrings, quadriceps, groin, gluteus, core, chest, spine, and shoulders.

Sports it benefits

REVOLVING HALF MOON BALANCE
(Parivrtta Ardha Chandrasana)

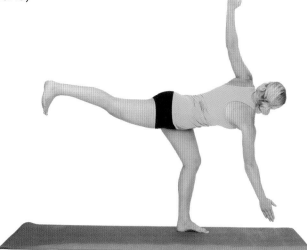

Let's see how far you can twist your Half Moon. This pose improves your sense of balance and coordination.

1. From Half Moon Balance pose, exhale and place your right hand on the floor next to your left foot.

2. Inhale and extend your left arm upward, while twisting your upper body to the left.

3. Ready? Lift your right hand 1 inch (2.5 cm) off the floor, and look at your left hand.

4. Press your left hip upward, while squeezing your left thigh. Take five to ten deep breaths, and repeat with your right foot on the floor.

Target body areas:

feet, ankles, calves, IT bands, hamstrings, quadriceps, groin, gluteus, core, obliques, chest, spine, and shoulders.

Sports it benefits

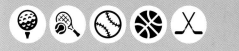

BALANCING BEAR

(Merudandasana)

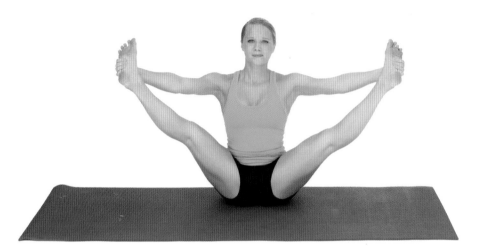

You may feel weird in this powerful pose, but I've actually seen grizzly bears do this in person. This pose provides a total core and balance workout.

1. Start in a seated position with your knees drawn toward you.

2. Grab your ankles or the outside of your feet, and extend your legs on a diagonal while activating your core.

3. Stretch your legs, arms, and chest as much as possible, while maintaining your balance and keeping your shoulders away from your ears. Hold for five to ten deep breaths, and release.

Target body areas:

hamstrings, inner thighs, hips, core, chest, wrists, and shoulders.

Sports it benefits

HANDSTAND
(Adho Mukha Vrksasana)

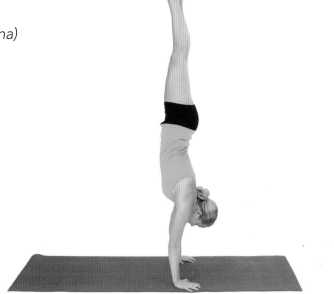

Handstand is a very challenging inversion and should only be attempted with caution and control.

1. Begin in Downward Facing Dog, and start slowly rocking forward and back to gain a little momentum.

2. Lift your left leg, while continuing to rock, and start activating your core. Start to add a hop to the rocking. Open your fingers wide, and relax your neck.

3. Swing your left leg up first followed by your right into a full handstand. Hold for five to ten deep breaths or as long as possible before slowly coming back down. Make sure to bend your knees when you land.

Modification: Practice your handstand against a wall or with a partner for extra support.

Target body areas:

quadriceps, core, hands, wrists, forearms, biceps, triceps, spine, and shoulders.

Sports it benefits

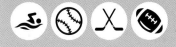

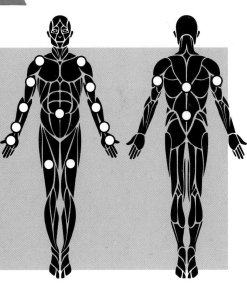

CHAPTER 4
WARRIORS

To be an athlete, you must train as a warrior. I've included a whole chapter of Warrior variations—well-known Warriors as well as new variations to keep you challenged and invigorated in your training. Warriors are very vigorous poses that demand strength and balance, while keeping your mind and body alert and ready for anything. In short, I feel a deep connection to my body and realize my true strength whenever I practice these poses. Even though I'm standing still, all my muscles are alert and active. You'll find all of the Warriors improve balance, focus, and posture. For full-body conditioning workout, flow through all fifteen of these in one routine. Find your inner warrior in this chapter.

WARRIOR 1

(Virabhadrasana I)

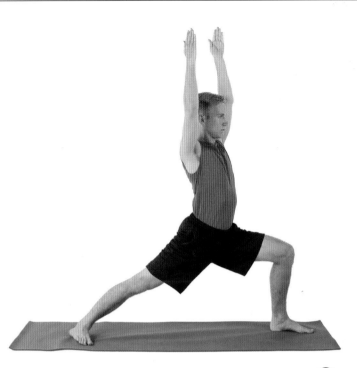

This pose opens the door to your true strength and balance and improves focus and stability.

1. From a standing position, step your left foot forward about 3 feet (0.9 m), and bend your left knee so it's directly above your ankle.

2. Turn your right foot out slightly so the heel touches the floor, and extend that leg.

3. Turn your upper body toward your left leg, and reach your arms overhead with your palms facing inward. Reach your fingers high, and relax your shoulders. Hold for five to ten deep breaths, and repeat with your right foot in front.

Target body areas:

ankles, quadriceps, hamstrings, hip flexors, abdominals, chest, biceps, triceps, back, and shoulders.

Sports it benefits

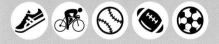

WARRIOR 2
(Virabhadrasana II)

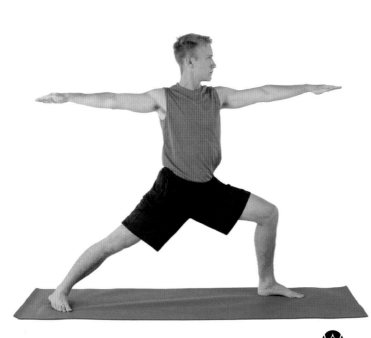

Nothing can improve your sense of inner power more than a Warrior.

1. From Warrior 1, drop your arms out to the sides so your upper body opens to the right.

2. Take your gaze forward, and look past the middle finger of your left hand.

3. Keep the posture of your legs the same, and keep stretching your back leg. Hold for five to ten deep breaths, and repeat with your right foot in front.

Target body areas:

ankles, quadriceps, hamstrings, hip flexors, abdominals, chest, biceps, triceps, back, and shoulders.

Sports it benefits

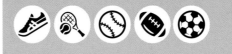

WARRIOR 3
(Virabhadrasana III)

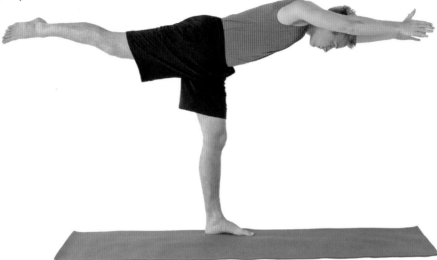

Welcome to the Warrior that brings along a whole lot of balance.

1. From Warrior 1, press your weight into your left (front) foot, and lift your back leg off the floor.

2. Extend your arms forward, and try to bring your body parallel to the floor, while keeping a little bend in your left leg.

3. Keep your chin tucked slightly, and activate your core. Find a spot on the floor in front of you to focus on. Hold for five to ten deep breaths, and repeat with your right foot in front.

Target body areas:

feet, ankles, calves, quadriceps, core, back, and shoulders.

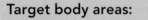

Sports it benefits

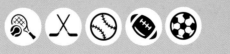

57

REVERSE WARRIOR

(Viparita Virabhadrasana)

Let's add some stretch to your Warrior.

1. From Warrior 1, inhale and reach your left arm up and into a backbend, while exhaling and sliding your right hand down your right leg.

2. Relax your shoulders, and stretch your back leg. Hold for five to ten deep breaths, and repeat with your right foot in front.

Target body areas:

ankles, quadriceps, hamstrings, hip flexors, abdominals, sides, back, and shoulders.

Sports it benefits

SIDE ANGLE WARRIOR

(Utthitaparsvakonasana)

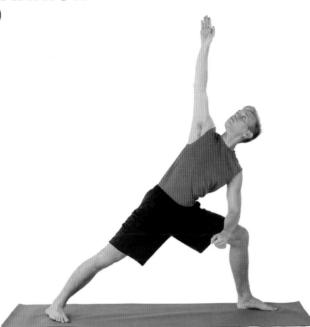

Were you missing a forearm aspect to your Warrior? Here it is.

1. From Reverse Warrior, exhale and bend your left arm, and place your forearm gently on your left thigh.

2. Inhale and reach your right arm upward, while pressing your right hip away and squeezing your back leg. Use your core to keep you lifted, not your forearm. Hold for five to ten deep breaths, and repeat with your right foot in front.

Target body areas:

ankles, quadriceps, hamstrings, hip flexors, core, chest, back, and shoulders.

Sports it benefits

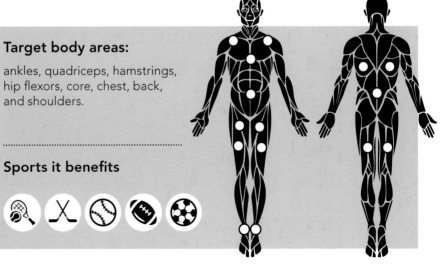

PROUD WARRIOR

(Utthita Parsvakonasana)

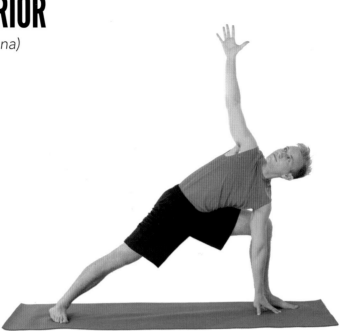

You should always feel great pride in adding Warriors to your life.

1. From Side Angle, place your left fingertips gently to the floor, draw your right shoulder back, and open your chest farther. Hold for five to ten deep breaths, and repeat with your right foot in front.

Target body areas:

ankles, quadriceps, hamstrings, hip flexors, core, chest, back, and shoulders.

Sports it benefits

WARRIOR WRAP

(Baddha Utthita Parsvakonasana)

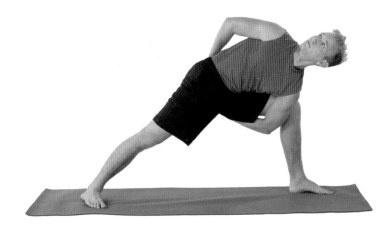

Wrap your way to some extreme flexibility and power.

1. From Proud Warrior, reach your left arm under your left thigh and your right arm around your lower back until they meet. Lace your fingers if possible.

2. Pull your right shoulder back, and open your chest as you stretch your right leg and take your eyes upward. Feeling it yet? Hold for five to ten deep breaths, and repeat with your right foot in front.

Modification: Just stay in Proud Warrior, and place your right arm on your lower back.

Target body areas:

ankles, quadriceps, hamstrings, hip flexors, core, chest, back, and shoulders.

Sports it benefits

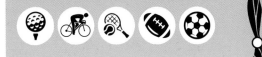

MUDRA WARRIOR

(Mudra Virabhadrasana)

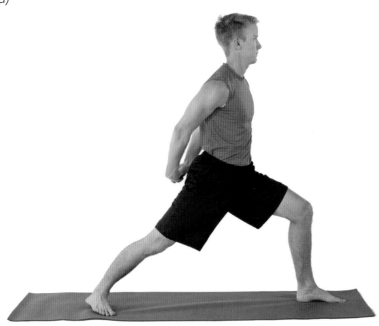

Get your posture fixed and your breath flowing with this pose.

1. From Warrior 1, bring your arms behind your back, and lace your fingers together.

2. Draw your shoulders down and back as you lengthen your arms and open your chest. Hold for five to ten deep breaths, and repeat with your right foot in front.

Target body areas:

ankles, quadriceps, hamstrings, hip flexors, abdominals, chest, back, and shoulders.

Sports it benefits

MUDRA WARRIOR 3
(Mudra Virabhadrasana III)

1. It's time to make that Mudra fly in this killer pose. From Mudra Warrior, place your weight into your left foot, and lift your right foot upward.

2. Take your eyes to the floor as you draw your arms back, and bring your body parallel to the floor. Keep a little softness in the left knee. Hold for five to ten deep breaths, and repeat with your right foot in front.

Target body areas:

feet, ankles, quadriceps, core, chest, back, and shoulders.

Sports it benefits

63

EAGLE WARRIOR

(Garudasana Viraghadrasana)

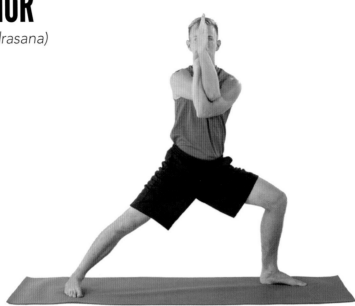

What happens when you combine Warrior with a heck of a lot of upper-body stretching? You get an upper-body stretch that also builds strength and balance in your lower body.

1. From Warrior 1, turn your upper body to the right.

2. Wrap your left arm under your right arm, and try to bring your palms together.

3. Draw your shoulders down, your elbows forward, and your fingers up. Hold for five to ten deep breaths, and repeat with your right foot in front.

Target body areas:

ankles, quadriceps, hamstrings, hip flexors, abdominals, chest, wrists, forearms, back, and shoulders.

Sports it benefits

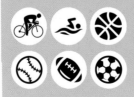

EAGLE WARRIOR 3
(Garudasana Viraghadrasana III)

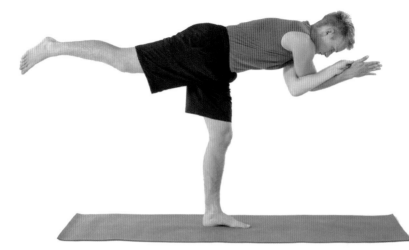

Let's test how well you can balance your Warrior.

1. From Eagle Warrior, turn your upper body forward, and place your weight onto your left foot.

2. Press forward so your right leg lifts off the floor, and try to bring yourself parallel to the floor.

3. Keep your eyes to the floor, and extend your elbows forward, while activating your core to stay centered. Hold for five to ten gloriously deep breaths, and repeat with your right foot in front.

Target body areas:

feet, ankles, calves, quadriceps, core, chest, wrists, forearms, back, and shoulders.

Sports it benefits

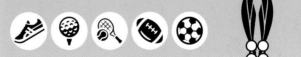

65

ARCHER WARRIOR

(Dhanurdhara Asana)

Grab your bow and arrow, and let's increase your willpower.

1. From Warrior 1, imagine you're holding a bow and arrow, and pull your right hand back as you hold the string and arrow.

2. Reach your left hand forward as you hold the bow. Line up your target as you flex your arms and shoulders before letting the arrow fly into your target. Hold for five to ten deep breaths, and repeat with your right foot in front.

Target body areas:

ankles, quadriceps, hamstrings, hip flexors, core, chest, biceps, triceps, back, and shoulders.

Sports it benefits

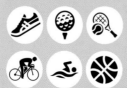

SIDE BEND WARRIOR
(Urdhva Hastasana Virabhadrasana)

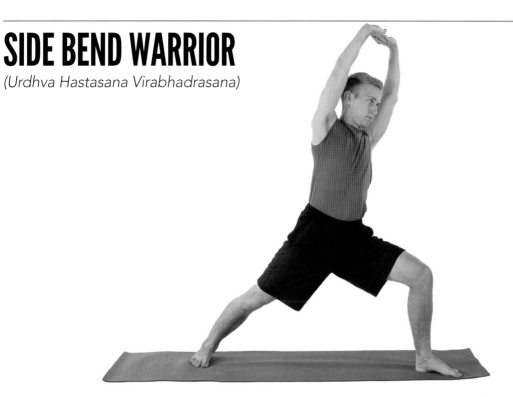

Open up and tone your obliques with this powerful Warrior.

1. From Warrior 1, lace your fingers together, and bend to the outside (left).

2. Inhale and lift your arms, and exhale as you bend farther. Feel the burn! Bend to the inside (right) and hold for five to ten deep breaths on both sides, then repeat while bending to the outside (left). Repeat with your right foot in front.

Target body areas:

ankles, quadriceps, hamstrings, hip flexors, core, obliques, sides, biceps, triceps, spine, back, and shoulders.

Sports it benefits

WARRIOR TWIST

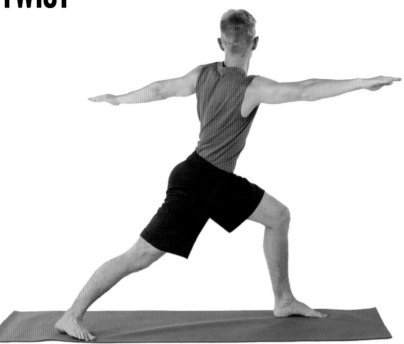

Only the strongest Warriors can twist with ease.

1. From Side Bend Warrior, inhale and extend your arms out to the sides in a straight line.

2. Exhale and twist your body to the outside (left) and hold. With each inhale, lift your body, and twist farther with each exhale. Hold for five to ten deep breaths and then twist to the inside (right). Repeat with your right foot in front.

Target body areas:

ankles, quadriceps, hamstrings, hip flexors, core, obliques, biceps, back, and shoulders.

Sports it benefits

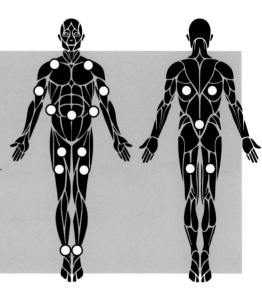

SPIDERMAN WARRIOR

(Spiderman Virabhadrasana)

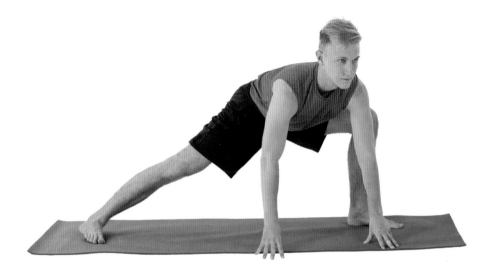

Scale walls, fight crime, and build a powerful body with an added spine stretch.

1. From Warrior Twist, walk your fingertips to the floor on your right, while keeping your back lengthened and your core engaged.

2. With each exhale, walk your fingers a little farther forward, while maintaining your powerful Warrior legs. Hold for five to ten deep breaths, watch out for criminals, and repeat with your right foot in front.

Target body areas:

ankles, quadriceps, hamstrings, hip flexors, core, obliques, biceps, triceps, back, and shoulders.

Sports it benefits

69

CHAPTER 5
STANDING

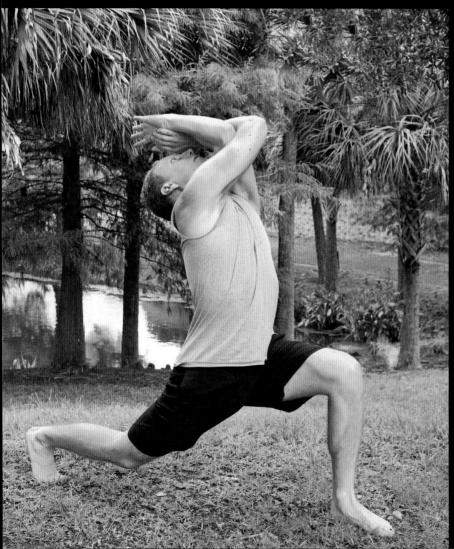

Stand and be strong! It's time to plant your feet on the ground and claim your strength with these essential standing poses. These poses will train your body as a whole to withstand any attack and bring strength, power, and resilience to your entire body. By mastering these poses, you'll be able to move quicker, more efficiently, and with great precision.

TRIANGLE

(Trikonasana)

These Triangle poses stimulate your abdominal organs, aiding in digestion.

1. Begin in a standing position, and step your left foot forward about 3 to 4 feet (0.9 to 1.2 m), opening your left hip and foot.

2. Turn your right foot in slightly, and raise your arms to the sides, while facing right with your upper body.

3. Inhale and extend left, then exhale and bring your left hand to the bottom of your left leg or the back of your hand to the inside of the ankle.

4. Press your right hip away, and inhale as you reach your right arm upward.

5. Keep drawing your right arm back, and look at your right hand, while squeezing your thighs. Hold for five to ten deep breaths, and repeat on the other side.

Modification: Place your left hand on your left thigh for more support.

Target body areas:

ankles, calves, hamstrings, groin, hips, abdominals, spine, back, and neck.

Sports it benefits

EXTREME TRIANGLE

(Trikonasana)

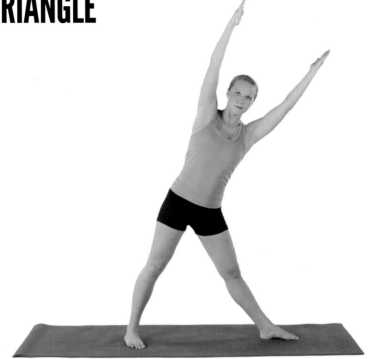

It's time to take our beloved Triangle to the extreme!

1. From Triangle pose, exhale and extend both arms to the left, while pressing your right hip farther to the right.

2. Inhale and draw your shoulders down, open your chest, and look into your armpit. Hold for five to ten deep breaths, and repeat on the other side.

Target body areas:

ankles, calves, hamstrings, groin, hips, core, obliques, chest, spine, back, neck, and shoulders.

Sports it benefits

REVERSE TRIANGLE

(Parivrtta Trikonasana)

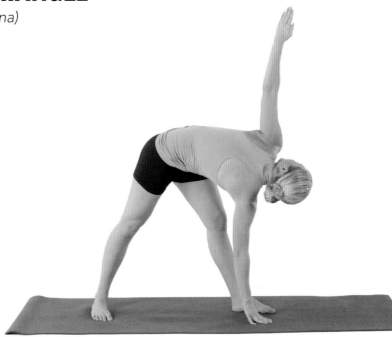

This pose feels great and really stretches the IT band.

1. From Extreme Triangle, exhale and reach your right hand to the floor next to your left foot.

2. Inhale and extend your left arm skyward as your upper body twists to the left.

3. Extend your left leg to really stretch that stubborn IT band. Hold for five to ten deep breaths, and repeat on the other side.

Modification: Place your right hand on your left leg for more support.

Target body areas:

ankles, calves, IT band, hamstrings, groin, hips, abdominals, obliques, spine, back, neck, and shoulders.

Sports it benefits

CRESCENT LUNGE

(Anjaneyasana)

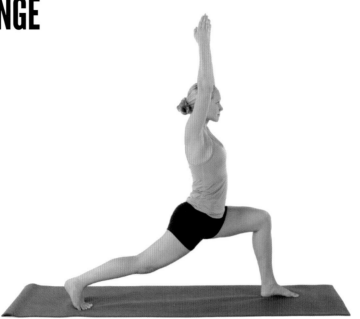

This classic Lunge will help you with any physical activity, improving stamina, balance, and focus.

1. From Triangle, turn your back foot forward, and bend your left leg 90 degrees so the knee is right above your ankle.

2. Inhale and reach both arms overhead, bringing your fingertips together.

3. Exhale as you press your right heel toward the floor, and inhale as you extend your fingers higher. So many muscles are having fun now! Hold for five to ten deep breaths, and repeat with your right foot in front.

Modification: Place your hands on your left thigh for more support.

Target body areas:

ankles, quadriceps, hip flexors, gluteus, core, and shoulders.

Sports it benefits

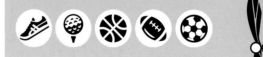

EAGLE LUNGE
(Garudasana Anjaneyasana)

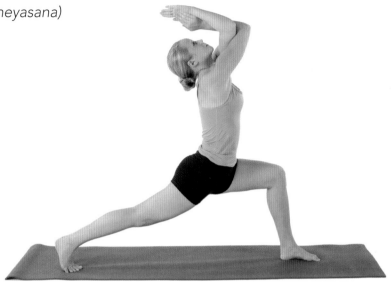

I say there's never too much Eagle, a pose that improves stamina, balance, and focus.

1. From Crescent Lunge, wrap your right arm under your left, and try to bring your palms together.

2. Inhale as you lift your fingers to the sky, and exhale as you sink lower into the lunge. Keep your chin tucked slightly and your jaw loose. Hold for five to ten heavenly breaths, and repeat with your right leg in front and your left arm under your right.

Target body areas:

ankles, quadriceps, hip flexors, gluteus, core, wrists, forearms, back, and shoulders.

Sports it benefits

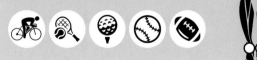

EAGLE LUNGE POINTER

(Garudasana Anjaneyasana)

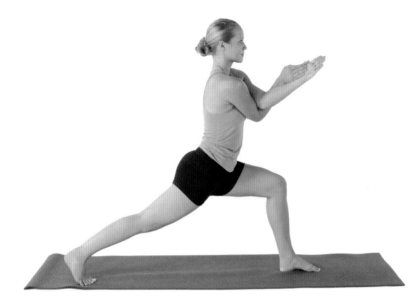

I may have invented this powerful and challenging pose. Patent pending! This one, too, improves stamina, balance, and focus.

1. From Eagle Lunge, exhale and pull your right elbow into your body.

2. Keep your back leg straight as you deepen the Eagle wrap. Hold for five to ten deep breaths, and repeat with your right leg in front and your left arm under your right.

Target body areas:

ankles, quadriceps, hip flexors, gluteus, core, wrists, forearms, back, and shoulders.

Sports it benefits

STANDING HALF MOON

(Ardha Chandrasana)

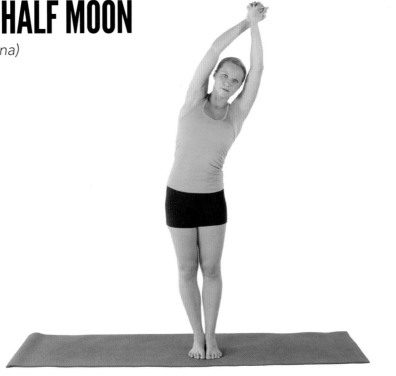

If you don't have a lot of space and need a loose spine, this pose is for you. It also improves focus and coordination.

1. From a standing position, bring your feet and legs together, and inhale as you bring your arms overhead and cross them, right behind left, lacing your fingers together.

2. Exhale and bend to your left, inhale and grow taller. Bend more to the left with each exhale.

3. Keep your shoulders back and down and your chest open. Hold for five to ten deep breaths, switch your hands, and repeat on the other side.

Target body areas:

feet, ankles, quadriceps, abdominals, obliques, sides, spine, and shoulders.

Sports it benefits

77

CHAIR TWIST
(Parivrtta Utkatasana)

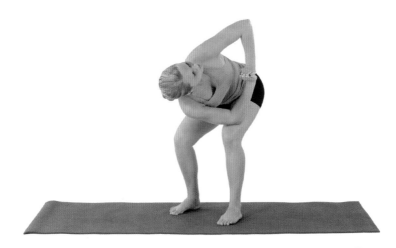

Take a seat, and give your core and legs a challenge they'll love!

1. From Chair pose, inhale and bring your palms together.

2. Exhale, twist your upper body to the left, and place your right arm gently on your left thigh.

3. Keep your knees together, and twist a little more with each exhale. Hold for five to ten deep breaths, and repeat on the other side.

Target body areas:

ankles, quadriceps, gluteus, core, obliques, biceps, triceps, and shoulders.

Sports it benefits

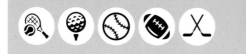

WIDE-LEGGED MUDRA

(Prasarita Padottasana)

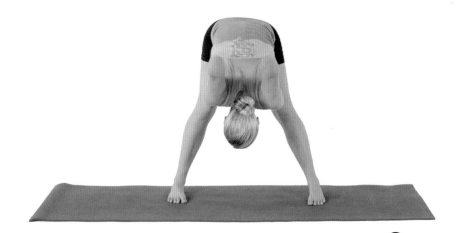

Fix your posture and stretch your legs in one powerful pose. This one brings lots of blood to the brain.

1. From a standing position, step your feet to a wide stance.

2. Inhale as you reach your arms behind you, and lace your fingers together.

3. Soften your knees, and exhale as you slowly dive toward the floor.

4. Put the weight into your toes, and draw your arms toward the back of your head with each exhale. Keep your head and neck relaxed. Hold for five to ten deep breaths, and slowly come back up.

Modification: Cross your arms on your lower back.

Target body areas:

ankles, Achilles tendon, calves, hamstrings, gluteus, lower back, spine, chest, and shoulders.

Sports it benefits

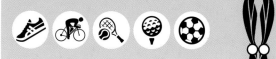

HALF MOON

(Ardha Chandrasana)

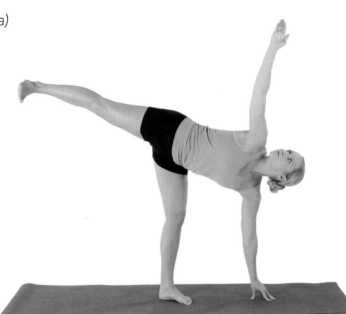

Here's another chance to enjoy Half Moon. This pose improves balance and coordination.

1. From Triangle pose, exhale and place your left hand on the floor about 1 foot (0.3 m) in front of your left foot.

2. Inhale and lift your right leg off the floor, while extending your right arm upward.

3. Roll your right shoulder back, and open your chest, while looking to your right hand. Hold for five to ten deep breaths, and repeat on the other side.

Target body areas:

ankles, calves, hamstrings, quadriceps, groin, gluteus, core, chest, spine, and shoulders.

....

Sports it benefits

REVOLVING HALF MOON

(Parivrtta Ardha Chandrasana)

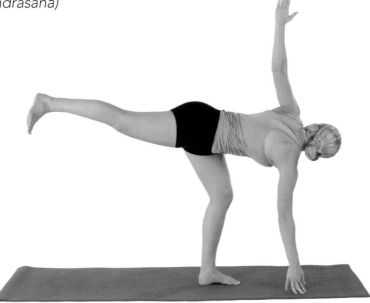

You've survived Half Moon. Now can you revolve it? This also improves balance and coordination.

1. From Half Moon, exhale and bring your right hand to the floor to the right of your right foot, inhale and extend your left hand upward.

2. Keep lifting your right leg, and take your eyes to your left hand. Feel the burn! Hold for five to ten deep breaths, and repeat on the other side.

Target body areas:

ankles, calves, IT bands, hamstrings, quadriceps, groin, gluteus, core, obliques, spine, chest, and shoulders.

Sports it benefits

81

STANDING SPLITS
(Urdhva Prasarvta Ekapadasana)

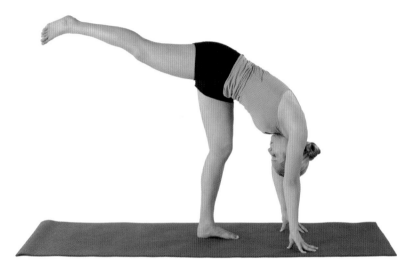

Can't do the splits? You can now do them while standing. This pose stimulates the liver and kidneys.

1. Begin in Triangle pose, exhale and press your weight forward, bringing your hands about 1 foot (0.3 m) in front of your left foot.

2. Exhale and lift your right leg off the floor. Tuck your chin, and keep lifting your right leg with each inhale. Hold for five to ten deep breaths, and repeat on your right foot.

Add-on: Bring both hands to your ankles for balance.

Target body areas:

ankles, calves, knees, hamstrings, quadriceps, gluteus, and core.

Sports it benefits

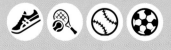

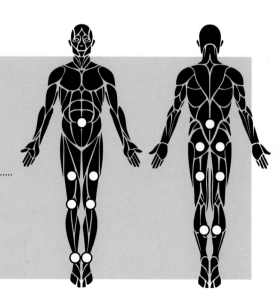

WIDE-CRESCENT LUNGE
(Anjaneyasana)

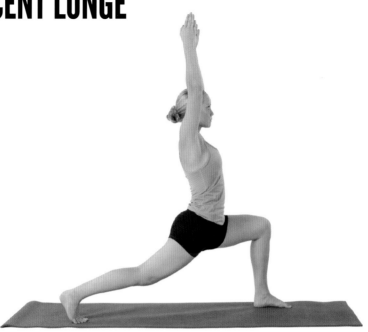

You can pull off the Crescent Lunge, but can you make it wide? This pose strengthens the quadriceps and gluteus, builds power and control in the core, stretches the lower back, and improves stamina, balance, and focus.

1. From Crescent Lunge, step your front foot (left) to the outside edge of your mat.

2. Feel the difference as you activate your core and lift your upper body tall with each inhale. Hold for five to ten deep breaths, and repeat with your right foot in front.

Target body areas:

quadriceps, hip flexors, gluteus, hips, and core.

Sports it benefits

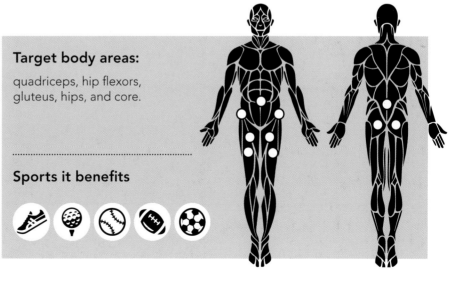

83

LUNGE TWIST

(Vakra Anjaneyasana)

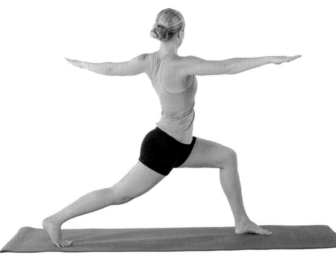

Any chance you get, add a twist to your poses! This pose strengthens the arms, legs, ankles, shoulders, and muscles of the back, stretches the sides and obliques, flattens and tones the core, and improves balance, focus, and posture.

1. From Crescent Lunge, inhale and extend your arms to the sides.

2. Exhale and twist your upper body to the outside (left) and keep your shoulders down. Hold for five to ten deep breaths, and repeat with your right foot in front.

Target body areas:

ankles, quadriceps, hamstrings, hip flexors, core, obliques, spine, biceps, triceps, back, and shoulders.

Sports it benefits

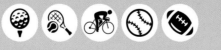

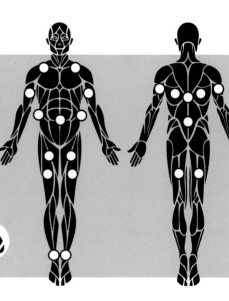

WALKING FORWARD FOLD

(Padangusthasana)

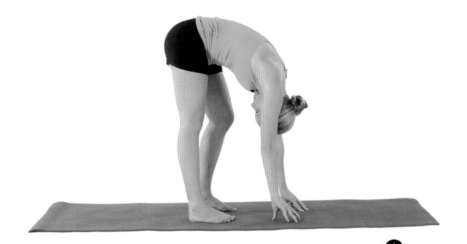

I teach this pose at the beginning of every class and with good reason. It calms the brain and helps relieve stress, stretches the hamstrings, calves, and hips, strengthens the thighs and knees, and helps reduce fatigue and anxiety.

1. From Mountain pose, soften your knees, and exhale as you slowly dive down toward your toes.

2. Put the weight in your toes as you slowly walk in place, while relaxing your neck and engaging your abs with each exhale. Walk for five to ten deep breaths, and slowly rise back up to standing.

Target body areas:

calves, knees, hamstrings, quadriceps, hips, and spine.

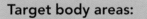

Sports it benefits

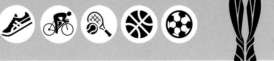

85

PLANKS

Finally, it's time for my favorite chapter: Planks! Anyone who knows me knows that I will drop down anywhere and anytime to do planks. I teach them in every class (even if it's spinning) and add them into pretty much every one of my more than 1,000 workout videos. Why this obsession? Planks work every ounce of your body and build power, strength, focus, and a rock-hard core. You can always place your forearms (instead of your hands) on the floor if you experience discomfort in your wrists. But, enough talking—let's get planking!

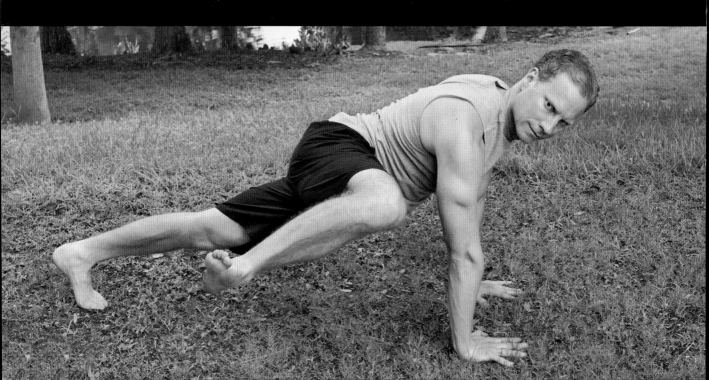

CLASSIC PLANK
(Dandasana)

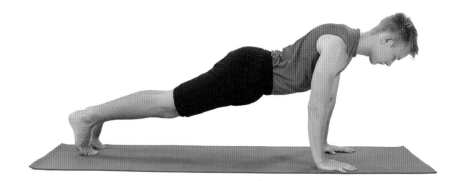

This is the original, can't-be-beat Classic Plank. Planks build total unity in the body. And Classic Plank is about to be your new best friend.

1. From hands and knees position, tuck your toes and lift your knees off the floor.

2. Place your hands under your shoulders, draw your shoulders back, tuck your chin slightly, and press through your heels. You're now Planking!

3. Flex your abs on every exhale for an extra burn. Hold for five to ten breaths.

Modification: You can always Plank with your knees down, but remember, the farther behind your hips you place the knees on the floor, the tougher the Plank.

Target body areas:

core, chest, wrists, biceps, triceps, spine, and shoulders.

Sports it benefits

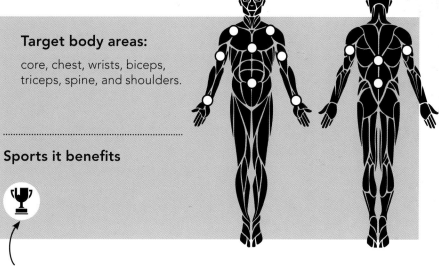

Note: You Plank, you excel. Whether you're marathon running or playing darts, these Planks will drastically improve your performance and strength in any physical endeavor.

FOREARM PLANK

(Phalakasana Forearm)

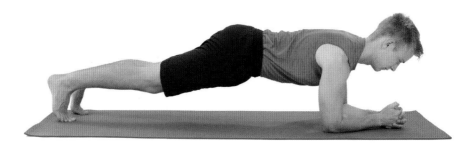

Here's the mighty brother of the Classic Plank if you're more of a forearm person. Remember: You can always Plank from your forearms if your wrists are bothering you.

1. From Classic Plank, drop your forearms down so the elbows are right under your shoulders.

2. Draw your shoulders and heels back, while squeezing your abs with each exhale. Don't forget to inhale! Hold for five to ten deep breaths, and bring your knees down.

Target body areas:

core, chest, wrists, biceps, triceps, spine, and shoulders.

Sports it benefits

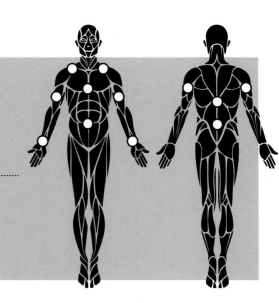

REVERSE PLANK
(Purvottanasana)

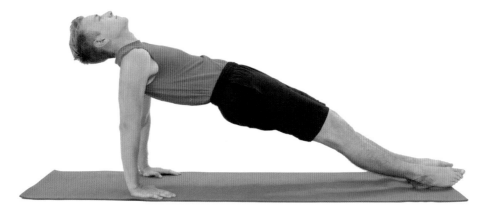

Tired of staring at the floor? Just flip your Plank on its back.

1. From a seated position, place your hands under your shoulders and point your feet.

2. Inhale and lift your bum and legs off the floor, while engaging your core. Find the hand position that works best.

3. Drop your shoulders back, and keep your neck in line with your spine. Hold for five to ten deep breaths.

Modification: Use your forearms instead, but I warn you—it's not much easier.

Target body areas:

hamstrings, gluteus, core, wrists, forearms, biceps, triceps, chest, and shoulders.

Sports it benefits

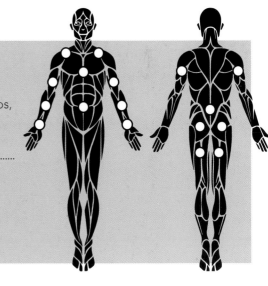

WALKOUT PLANK

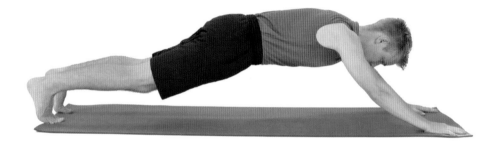

This plank can move!

1. From Classic Plank, walk your hands in front of your shoulders to a spot you can maintain.

2. Squeeze your abs on the exhales, and draw your shoulders back. It burns, doesn't it? Hold for five to ten deep breaths, and gently bring your knees down.

Target body areas:

core, chest, wrists, forearms, biceps, triceps, spine, back, and shoulders.

....

Sports it benefits

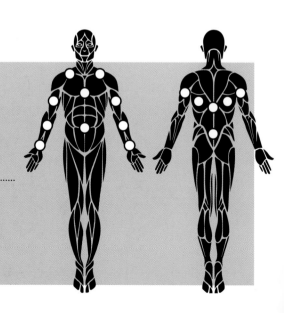

SIDE PLANK
(Vasisthasana)

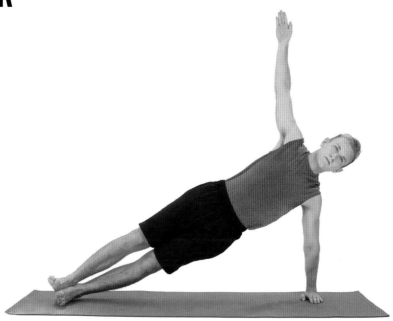

You can use Planks to really target and tone your sides and harden your core. It also improves balance.

1. From Classic Plank, inhale and lift your right arm up into a "T" shape.

2. Make sure your standing hand (left) is under your shoulder. Look up to your right hand. Hold for five to ten deep breaths, and repeat on the other side.

Target body areas:

quadriceps, hamstrings, core, obliques, wrists, forearms, biceps, and triceps.

Sports it benefits

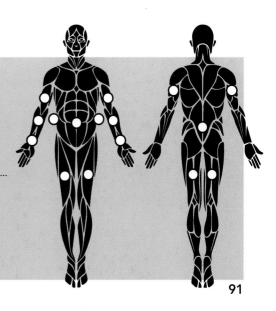

WIDE PLANK

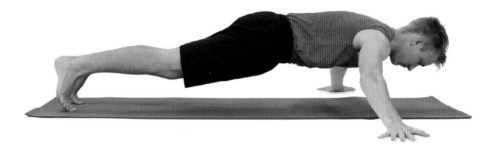

I've used this bad boy in some of my videos, and it really makes my muscles shake!

1. From Classic Plank, walk your hands to the outside as far as possible, while maintaining a parallel body.

2. Point your fingers to the outside, and keep a little softness in your elbows. Try to hold it for five to ten deep breaths, or as long as possible, and know you're building a strong, powerful, and athletic body.

Target body areas:

core, back, chest, wrists, forearms, biceps, triceps, spine, and shoulders.

Sports it benefits

ONE-ARMED PLANK

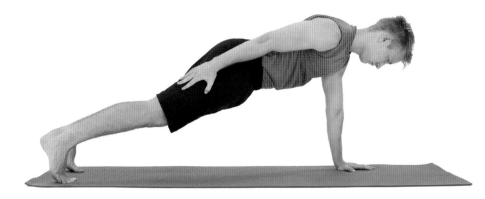

By lifting an arm from the Classic Plank, you open up your core to a whole new challenging level.

1. From Classic Plank, lift your right arm to your right side, and hold for five to ten deep breaths before repeating on the other side. That's it!

Target body areas:

core, chest, wrists, forearms, biceps, triceps, spine, and shoulders.

Sports it benefits

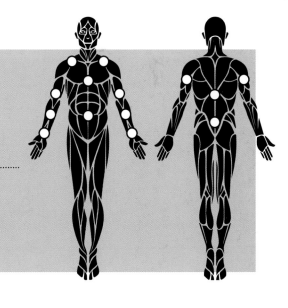

HOVER PLANK

(Chaturanga Dandasana)

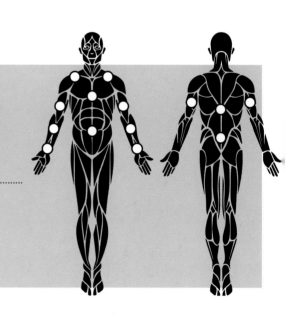

When you're ready to take your Plank to the next level, it's time to hover.

1. From Classic Plank, pull your elbows into your side, and exhale as you slowly lower down to about 5 inches (12.7 cm) off the floor.

2. Pull your shoulders back, press through your heels, and tuck your chin as the sweat begins to fall. Hold for five to ten deep breaths, and slowly rise back to Plank (or collapse).

Target body areas:

core, chest, wrists, forearms, biceps, triceps, spine, and shoulders.

....

Sports it benefits

CAT PLANK
(Marjaryasana Kumbhakasana)

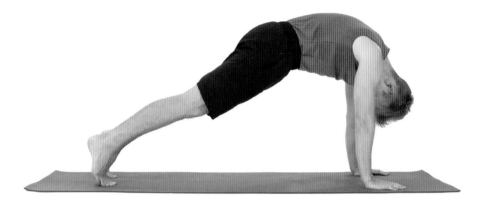

Let's add a total spine stretch to your Plank.

1. From Classic Plank, inhale, press your weight forward, and round your upper back upward.

2. Tuck your chin, and let your shoulders go slightly in front of your hands. Hold for five to ten deep breaths, and release. Meow.

Target body areas:

core, chest, wrists, forearms, biceps, triceps, spine, and shoulders.

Sports it benefits

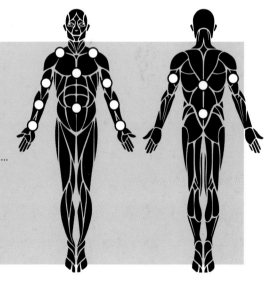

FROZEN SPIDERMAN PLANK

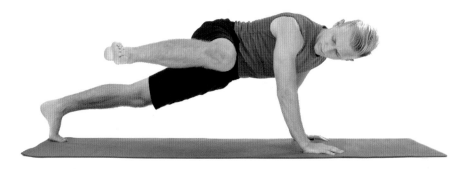

No, it's not a drink, but you may want one after doing this unique Plank.

1. From Classic Plank, exhale and pull your right knee toward your side.

2. Keep your leg lifted, and flex your foot. Hold for five to ten deep breaths, and repeat on the other side. Go, Plank, go!

Target body areas:

gluteus, hips, core, chest, wrists, forearms, biceps, triceps, spine, and shoulders.

Sports it benefits

FROZEN DOOR SWING PLANK

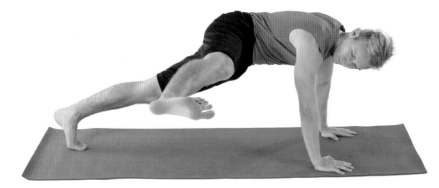

Once you've mastered the Spiderman, it's time to open the door.

1. From Frozen Spiderman Plank, exhale and extend your leg as far as possible to the side.

2. Take your eyes to that leg, and hold for five to ten deep breaths. Repeat on both sides.

Target body areas:

hips, gluteus, core, chest, wrists, forearms, biceps, triceps, spine, and shoulders.

Sports it benefits

LEG LIFT PLANK

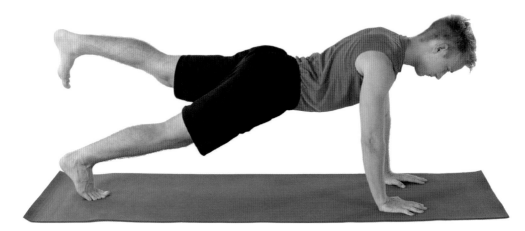

This may sound simple, but the real challenge is not letting your leg lower even one-tenth of an inch.

1. From Classic Plank, inhale and lift your left leg without moving any other part of your body. Flex your foot to engage your calf. Hold for five to ten deep breaths, and repeat on the other side.

Target body areas:

calves, hips, gluteus, core, chest, wrists, forearms, biceps, triceps, spine, and shoulders.

Sports it benefits

POPEYE PLANK

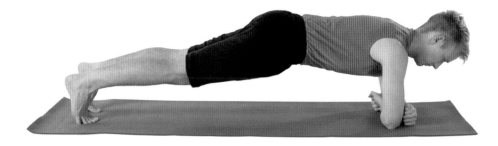

Get the strength of Popeye without having to gorge on spinach.

1. From Classic Plank, stack your forearms with the elbows under the shoulders, and tuck your toes.

2. Draw your shoulders back, flex your guns (arms and shoulders), and press your heels back. Hold for five to ten deep breaths, and slowly release.

Target body areas:

hips, core, chest, wrists, forearms, biceps, triceps, spine, and shoulders.

Sports it benefits

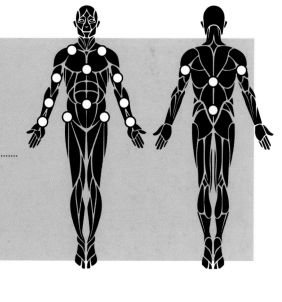

POPEYE TAP PLANK

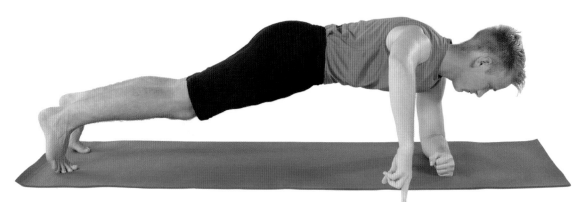

Popeye is best when he's moving. This pose builds total stamina, unity, and balance in the body.

1. From Popeye Plank, inhale and extend your right arm to the right side.

2. Gently place your fingertips on the floor, and hold for five to ten deep breaths. Repeat on the other side.

Target body areas:

hips, gluteus, core, chest, wrists, biceps, triceps, spine, and shoulders.

Sports it benefits

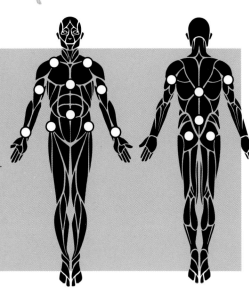

TABLE TOP PLANK

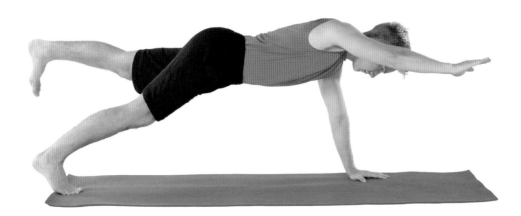

Less than 1 percent of my clients can really nail this plank. It requires incredible core stamina coupled with a laser-beam focus and balance.

1. From Classic Plank, inhale and extend your left leg and right arm. Try to hold for at least two breaths before switching to the other side.

2. Go back and forth ten times, and focus on lowering slowly. You can also hold each side for five to ten deep breaths to build incredible stamina. Good luck!

Target body areas:

hips, gluteus, core, chest, wrists, forearms, biceps, triceps, spine, and shoulders.

Sports it benefits

CHAPTER 7
CORE

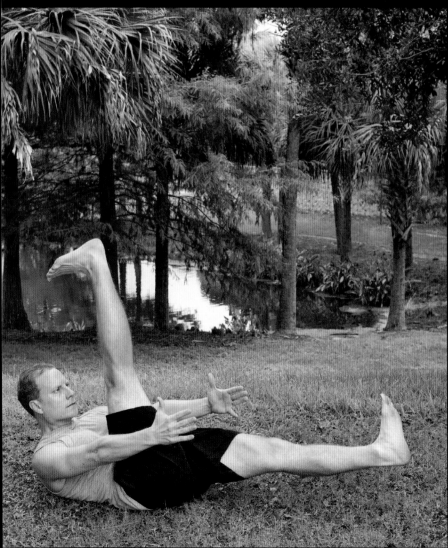

Many people don't realize that yoga is full of poses that will help you build that strong and powerful core (abdominals, hips, gluteus, and lower back). Every movement your body makes, either begins or passes through your core. It also supports your spinal column and connects your upper and lower body together. Without proper core strength, your body becomes very inefficient and will compensate by putting undue stress on other parts of your body, creating imbalances. This chapter contains poses that require no equipment or machines and can travel with you on the road. It's my pleasure to share with you these poses that will add speed, power, and control to your body—and make your competition scared to death.

REACH FOR THE SKY

This pose, with the great view of the sky, really digs deep into your core.

1. Lie on your back and inhale. Extend your legs to the sky.

2. With your legs about 3 to 5 inches (7.6 to 12.7 cm) apart, exhale and lift your head and shoulders off the mat, and reach your fingers straight up. Flex your feet for a deeper burn. Hold five to ten deep breaths, and slowly release.

Modification: Keep your knees bent.

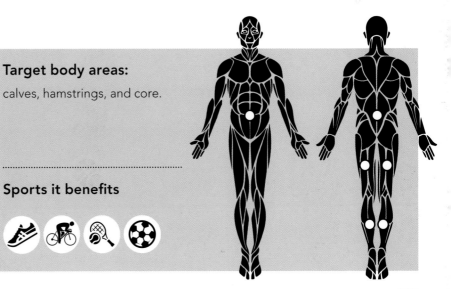

Target body areas:

calves, hamstrings, and core.

Sports it benefits

FROZEN SCISSORS

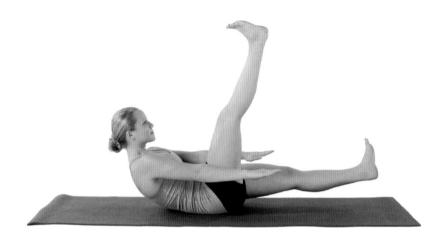

This is one of my "finishing" moves in my power yoga classes to squeeze every drop of weakness from our core. Don't be afraid if your body shakes; it means you're recruiting and building new muscles.

1. From Reach for the Sky, exhale and extend your left leg forward.

2. Inhale and extend your arms forward. Hold for five to ten deep breaths, while squeezing your abs with each exhale. Flex your feet for more core joy, and repeat on both sides.

Modificaion: Bend your knees.

Target body areas:

calves, hamstrings, quadriceps, and core.

Sports it benefits

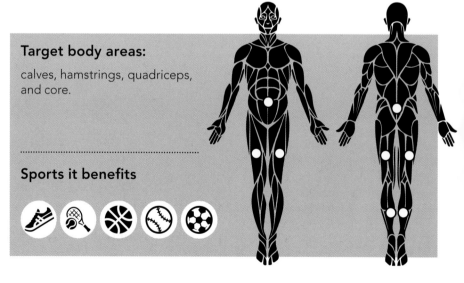

CRAB
(Catuspadapitham)

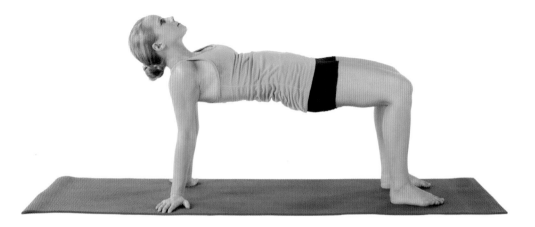

I love crab legs, but I love the core and gluteus toning of Crab pose even more. Crab also stimulates the respiratory and endocrine systems.

1. From a seated position, place your hands on the floor behind you, inhale and press up so your hands are above your wrists. Lengthen your arms fully with a slight bend in your elbows. Find the hand position that feels best.

2. Walk your heels below your knees, and squeeze your abs with each exhale to keep your core tight. Imagine there's a cactus underneath your bum, and keep your center lifted. Keep your chin slightly tucked, and hold for five to ten deep breaths.

Modification: If you have wrist issues, place your forearms down instead.

Target body areas:

quadriceps, hamstrings, core, chest, wrists, forearms, biceps, and triceps.

Sports it benefits

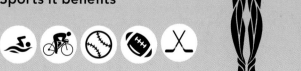

105

BALANCE THE CAT

(Dvitiya Bidala Tulana)

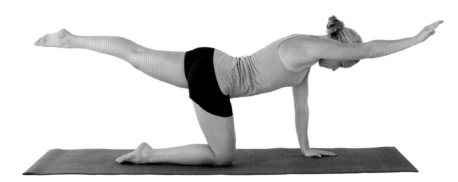

I've never seen a cat actually do this pose, but humans really love what it does for their core strength, focus, and balance.

1. From hands and knees position, inhale and extend your left leg behind you and your right arm in front.

2. Keep your body parallel to the floor, your chin slightly tucked, and your abs squeezing with each exhale. Hold for five to ten deep breaths before switching sides.

Target body areas:

gluteus, core, wrists, forearms, biceps, triceps, and shoulders.

Sports it benefits

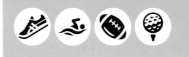

AWKWARD AIRPLANE

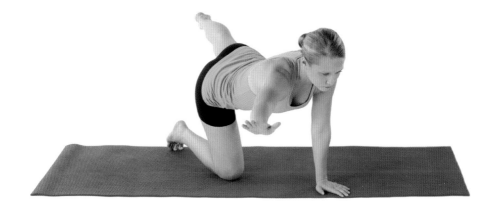

Awkward yes, but fantastic for core balance and gluteus toning. This pose builds balance throughout the body and focuses energy.

1. From Balance the Cat, inhale and extend your arm and leg on a diagonal to engage your gluteus and core on a deeper level. It's beautifully awkward! Hold for five to ten deep breaths, and repeat on the other side.

Target body areas:

gluteus, core, wrists, forearms, biceps, triceps, and shoulders.

Sports it benefits

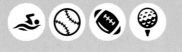

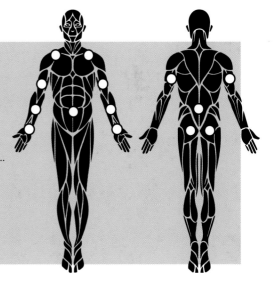

NOSE TO KNEE CRUNCH

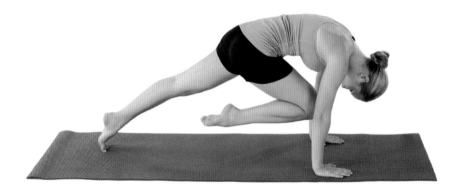

Nose, meet knee. Knee, meet nose. Core, prepare to work.

1. From Classic Plank, exhale and pull your right knee toward your chest as you round your back and squeeze your abs.

2. Pull your shoulders back as you hold this tough pose for five to ten deep breaths, and repeat with the other leg.

Target body areas:

core, wrists, forearms, biceps, triceps, spine, and shoulders.

Sports it benefits

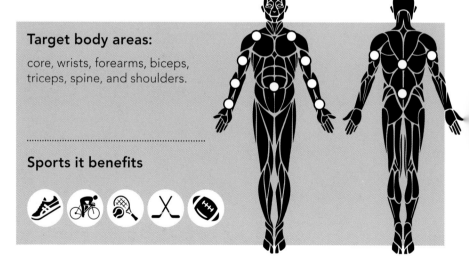

HALF BOAT

(Ardha Navasana)

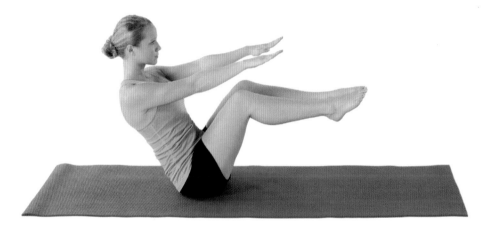

Let's pull anchor and set sail in search of a well-built core and better posture. This pose builds balance and focus.

1. From a seated position, walk your feet toward your gluteus, and roll your shoulders back and down, while opening your chest.

2. As you inhale, lift your feet off the floor, and bring them together directly in front of your knees, keeping them bent. Extend your arms with your palms down to your sides.

3. Tuck your chin slightly, and squeeze your abs on each exhale. Hold for five to ten deep breaths. Bon voyage!

Modification: You may gently hold onto your legs for more support or just keep your feet on the floor.

Target body areas:

hip flexors, core, and shoulders.

Sports it benefits

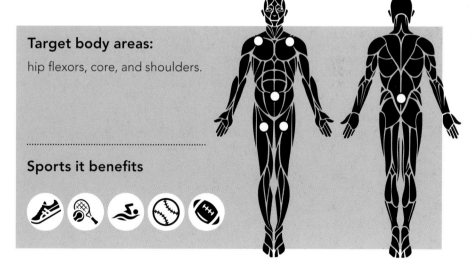

FULL BOAT

(Navasana)

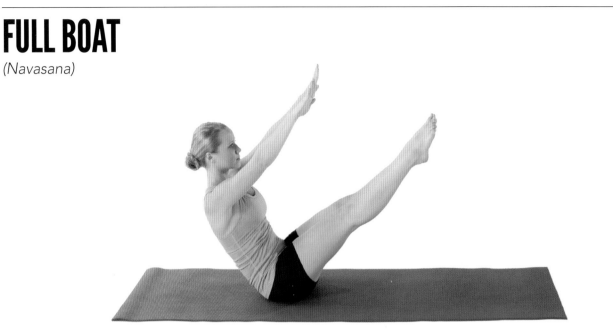

Once you get the hang of yoga boating, try going into deeper water and really constructing a powerful core. This pose helps correct posture and builds balance and focus.

1. From Half Boat, inhale and extend your legs on a diagonal.

2. Keep your arms to the sides, or raise them over your head to really feel this pose. Hold for five to ten deep breaths, and then hit the shore.

Target body areas:

quadriceps, hip flexors, core, back, and shoulders.

Sports it benefits

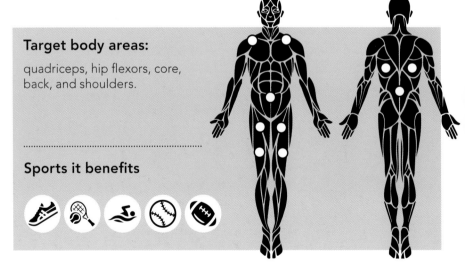

EAGLE BOAT

(Garudasana Navasana)

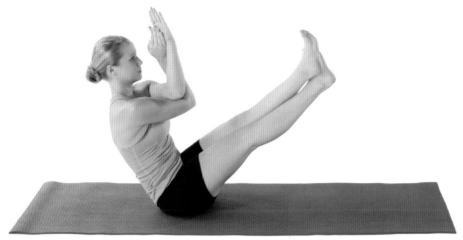

If you follow my YouTube page, you know I'll add the powerful Eagle to just about anything because of the combo of shoulder and chest stretching.

1. From Half Boat, inhale and wrap your right arm under and around your left arm for Eagle arms.

2. Exhale and cross your left leg over your right. You can also extend your legs into Full Boat and cross from there.

3. Inhale and reach your fingers to the sky as you exhale and squeeze your abs. Feel those muscles working! Hold for five to ten deep breaths, and release.

Target body areas:

quadriceps, hip flexors, core, wrists, forearms, back, and shoulders.

Sports it benefits

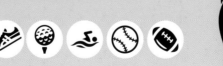

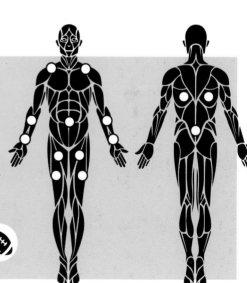

111

EXTENDED BOAT

(Paripuma Navasana)

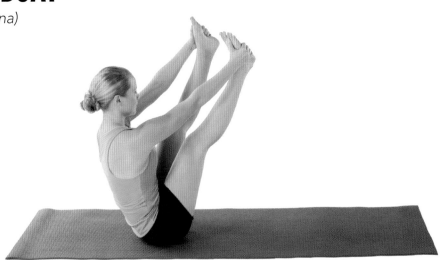

Now we're going to add a massive hamstring stretch to your boat practice.

1. From Half Boat, grab your ankles, and inhale as you extend your legs up to the sky.

2. On the next inhale, soften the knees slightly, and continue to extend on the exhale. Find your balance, and grab your feet if possible. This is an extremely powerful pose that will enhance your performance on every level. Hold for five to ten deep breaths, and release slowly.

Modification: Grab the backs of your legs, and draw your knees toward your chest. With each exhale, extend your legs a little more, and work your way up.

Target body areas:

hamstrings, inner thighs, core, wrists, back, and shoulders.

....

Sports it benefits

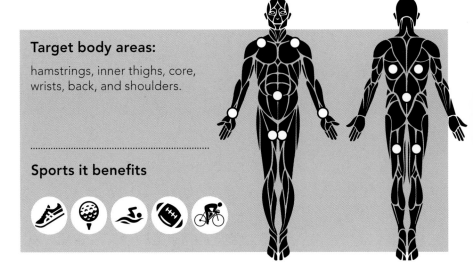

WIDE-LEGGED BOAT

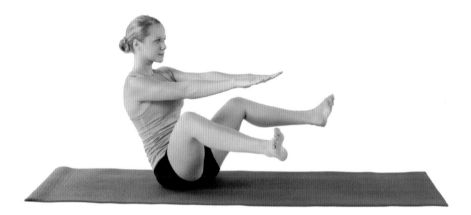

Say hello to your hips with this unique Boat variation. This pose builds tremendous balance and focus and is a great posture corrector.

1. From Half Boat, inhale and open your hips wider to a comfortable spot. Flex your feet.

2. Exhale and extend your arms forward between your legs. Hold for five to ten deep breaths, and slowly release.

Modification: Place your hands on your legs for more support.

Target body areas:

calves, inner thighs, hip flexors, gluteus, core, back, and shoulders.

Sports it benefits

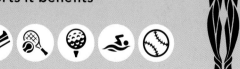

EXTREME BOAT

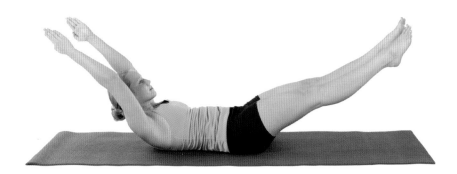

Alas, the final Boat is upon us. I saved the most extreme core blast for last. This pose builds power and endurance.

1. From Half Boat, exhale and slowly lower your back to the floor.

2. Inhale and extend your arms overhead, while lengthening your legs and dropping them as close to the floor as possible.

3. Keep your lower back on the floor at all times, and hold for five to ten deep breaths. Shaking is normal!

Modification: Bend your knees, or bring your head to the floor. You may also bring your arms to your sides instead.

Target body areas:

quadriceps, hip flexors, core, back, and shoulders.

Sports it benefits

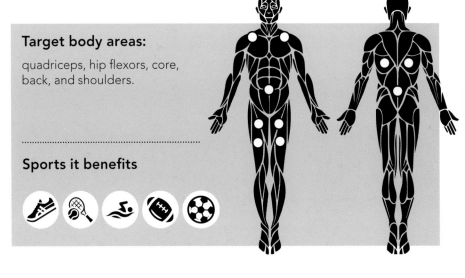

SUPERMAN
(Viparita Shalabhasana)

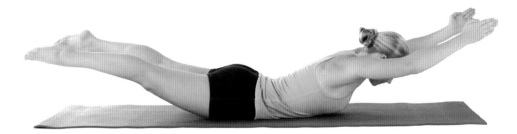

Superman pose (also great for a Superwoman) is a super way to work your lower back and abs. It also improves blood circulation and posture.

1. Begin on your stomach, and extend your arms forward. Make sure your arms are shoulder-width apart and your legs are hip-width apart.

2. Inhale and lift your arms and legs off the mat, while keeping your eyes to the floor.

3. Exhale and lengthen from your fingertips to the tips of your toes. Hold for five to ten deep breaths, and release.

Target body areas:

quadriceps, hamstrings, gluteus, core, biceps, triceps, chest, and shoulders.

Sports it benefits

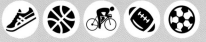

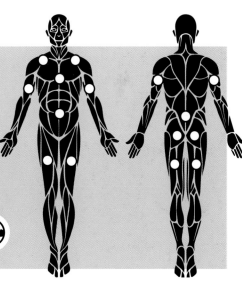

SHOULDER BRIDGE/WHEEL

(Setu Bandhasana/Urdhva Dhanurasana)

From Boat to Bridge—let's keep your core, back, and gluteus working! This pose increases energy.

1. From Extreme Boat, exhale and place your heels under your knees on the floor and your arms to your sides.

2. Inhale, tilt your pelvis up, and slowly lift off the floor into Shoulder Bridge. Feel the weight in your shoulders. Lace your fingers together and hold for five to ten deep breaths, before exhaling and slowly lowering down.

3. Let's talk Wheel pose. Place your hands on the floor like you're going into a gymnastic backbend, inhale and press skyward, while lifting your hips and engaging your quadriceps. Hold for five to ten deep breaths, and slowly return to earth.

Target body areas:

quadriceps, hamstrings, gluteus, core, spine, chest, wrists, forearms, biceps, triceps, and shoulders.

Sports it benefits

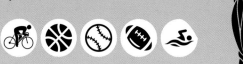

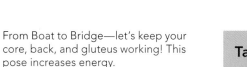

WIDE-LEGGED TWIST
(Prasarita Padottanasana)

Let's get off the floor for our final Core pose, which is also a fantastic twist.

1. Come to a standing wide-legged position with your toes pointed forward.

2. Exhale and place your left hand on the floor directly below your chest.

3. Inhale and lift your right arm skyward. Stay parallel to the floor, hold for five to ten deep breaths, and repeat on the other side.

Target body areas:

ankles, calves, hamstrings, inner thighs, obliques, chest, and shoulders.

Sports it benefits

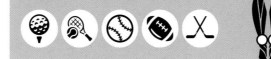

117

CHAPTER 8
COOL DOWN AND STRETCH

Finally, you've earned this, my friends! In power yoga, we take our cool-downs very seriously because they allow the cardiovascular system to slowly return to normal functioning, increase flexibility, lengthen muscles, and give your mind a chance to release and focus on each breath. The more you stretch and keep your body pliable, the younger you will feel and the more resistant to injury you'll be. Here are some of my favorites to make sure you're always feeling youthful, strong, and ready for the next challenge. Some of these entries include two or three poses, and one leads right into the next for optimum performance results.

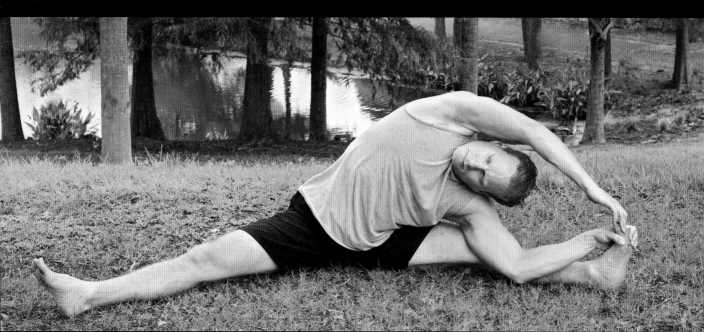

CHILD'S POSE/THREAD THE NEEDLE

(Balasana/Suci Sutrana)

There's a reason why children are naturally flexible. This combo calms the brain and helps relieve stress and fatigue.

1. From hands and knees position, exhale and slide your hands forward as you press your tailbone back.

2. Relax your neck, walk your fingers forward with each exhale, and draw your shoulders back with each inhale. Ahh, so nice. Hold for five to ten deep breaths.

3. To add Thread the Needle, exhale and slide your left arm under your right, bringing your face all the way to the floor.

4. Keep your eyes on your left hand. Hold for five to ten deep breaths, and repeat on the other side.

Target body areas:

ankles, quadriceps, obliques, lower back, and shoulders.

Sports it benefits

119

LOW LUNGE/SPLITS

(Anjaneyasana/Hanumanasana)

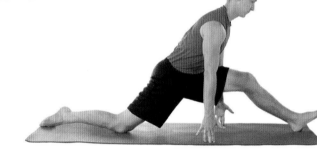

Have you always wanted to do the splits? This sequence is a great place to start.

1. From Crescent Lunge, exhale and lower your back knee, and place your hands on the floor.

2. Pull yourself slowly forward to stretch your quadriceps and hip flexors. Hold for five to ten deep breaths, and repeat on the other side.

3. Ready to move into the Splits? Exhale and slowly extend your front leg forward, making sure to keep your hands on the floor for support. Move slowly and cautiously with your breath. Hold for five to ten deep breaths, and repeat on the other side.

Target body areas:

calves, knees, hamstrings, quadriceps, hip flexors, and groin.

Sports it benefits

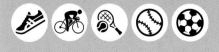

FOLDING LEAF/CROSS-LEGGED FOLDING LEAF

(Paschimottanasana)

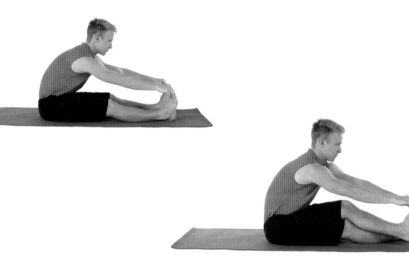

These are a couple of leaves that will bring lots of release to your spine and hamstrings.

1. From a seated position, exhale and extend your legs forward at hip-width.

2. Inhale, lift your arms overhead, and exhale as you hinge forward, grabbing your toes, feet, or ankles. Hold for five to ten deep breaths, and stay lifted instead of dropping down on your legs.

3. To get to Cross-Legged Folding Leaf, simply cross your left ankle over your right, and repeat the process for five to ten deep breaths, then repeat on the other side. This is a *great* IT band stretch!

Target body areas:

Achilles tendon, calves, IT bands, hamstrings, lower back, and spine.

Sports it benefits

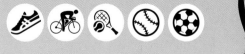

STRADDLE/STRADDLE TWIST/SIDE BEND STRADDLE

(Upavistha Konasana)

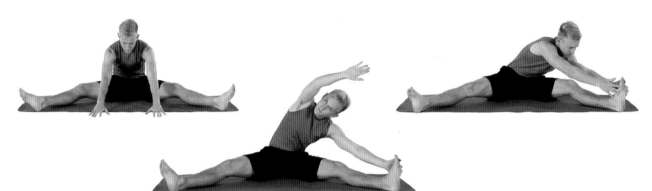

This is my post-workout go-to total-body stretch series. Hold all three for five to ten breaths. Do this routine after every practice, workout, and class to see and feel major differences.

1. From a seated position, inhale and open your legs as wide as is comfortable.

2. Exhale and hinge your upper body forward with your arms leading the way.

3. Inhale, lift slightly, and exhale as you hinge farther forward.

4. To add Straddle Twist, inhale and lift your upper body, then exhale and lengthen over your left leg. Repeat on both sides.

5. To add Side Bend Straddle, inhale and extend your left arm upward.

6. Exhale and lengthen your upper body into a side bend, trying to touch your right leg or foot. Repeat on both sides.

Target body areas:

ankles, calves, hamstrings, inner thighs, groin, hips, core, obliques, and shoulders.

Sports it benefits

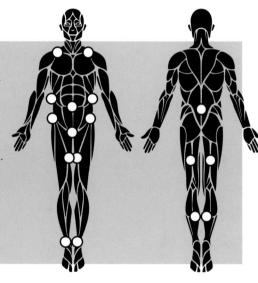

SPIDER
(Supta Padangustasana)

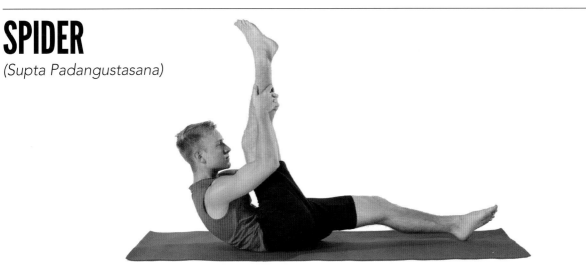

The only thing scary about this Spider is how much your hamstrings love it! Every athlete needs loose hamstrings to compete at 100 percent.

1. Lie on your back, and inhale as you extend your right leg upward.

2. Inhale and grab your leg as high as possible. Lift your head and shoulders off the floor.

3. Inhale, bend your knees slightly, and exhale as you extend the leg. Hold for five to ten deep breaths, and repeat on the other leg.

Modification: You may keep your head on the floor.

Target body areas:

ankles, calves, hamstrings, and lower back.

Sports it benefits

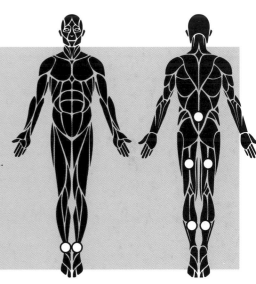

HAPPY BABY

(Ananda Balasana)

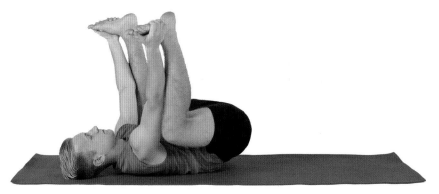

The other name for this massive hip opener is the "Dead Bug." It provides a nice lower back massage.

1. Lie on your back, and grab the insides or outsides of your feet with the inhale.

2. Exhale and open your hips while keeping your knees bent. Imagine your knees are very heavy.

3. Rock slowly side to side as you massage your lower back into the floor and open your hips. Hold for five to ten deep breaths.

Target body areas:

calves, knees, inner thighs, hips, and lower back.

Sports it benefits

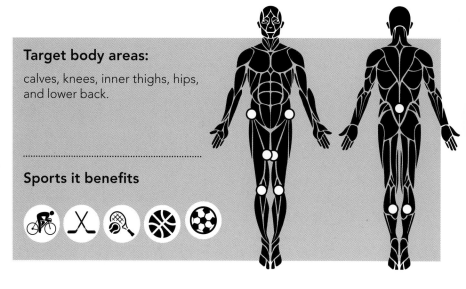

124

LYING SPINAL TWIST

(Supta Matsyendrasana)

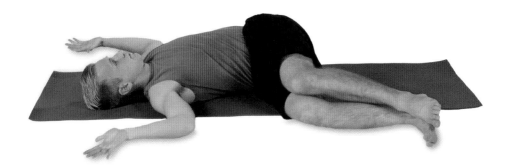

This is the pose I assign most as homework to my clients. Do it every morning and night! It even aids in digestion and helps with anxiety.

1. Lie on your back, inhale, and pull your knees into your chest.

2. Exhale and draw both legs to your right into a full twist.

3. Take your eyes to your left arm, and relax with each exhale. You may also grab the bottom foot with your left hand for a bigger stretch. Hold for five to ten deep breaths, and repeat on the other side. Your spine loves you for doing this.

Target body areas:

IT bands, hips, lower back, spine, back, chest, and shoulders.

Sports it benefits

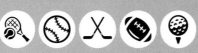

125

HURDLE
(Janu Sirsasana)

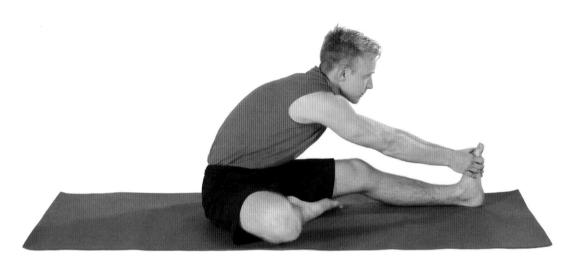

I would perform this move when running track, and it really made me run faster.

1. From a seated position, exhale and extend your left leg forward, and draw your right foot to your inner thigh.

2. Inhale as you lift your arms overhead and hinge up and over your left leg. Hold for five to ten deep breaths, and repeat on the other leg.

Target body areas:

calves, hamstrings, hips, lower back, and spine.

Sports it benefits

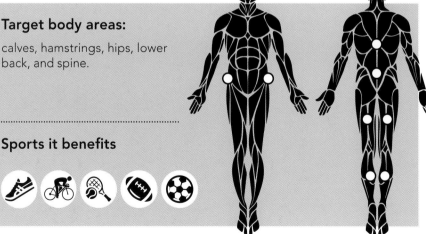

RUNNER'S STRETCH/PYRAMID
(Parsvottanasana)

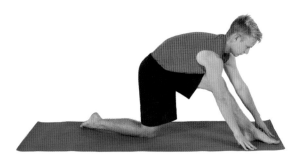

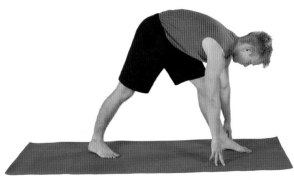

You may think these are only for runners, but they're for anyone who wants to run faster. Hold both poses for five to ten deep breaths, and repeat on both sides. This stretch improves posture and balance.

1. From Low Lunge, inhale and lengthen your front leg (left), while placing your right knee under your right hip.

2. Exhale and hinge forward, while bringing your hands to the floor.

3. Adding Pyramid will take this stretch up a notch! Tuck your right foot, and extend your right leg to add a deeper stretch from front to back. Place your hands on your leg or the floor, and lengthen over the front leg with every exhale.

Target body areas:

calves, hamstrings, quadriceps, spine, and shoulders.

Sports it benefits

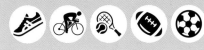

CAT/COW
(Marjaryasana)

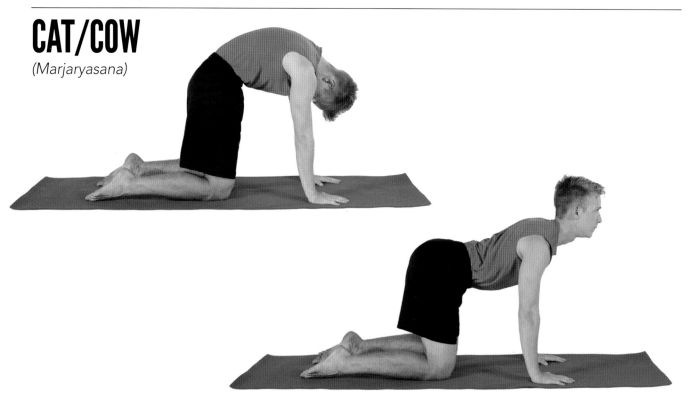

There's a wonderful spine stretch in this peculiar pairing of animals. It releases tension and anxiety throughout the body and spine.

1. From hands and knees position, for Cat, inhale and round your upper back to the sky, while dropping your head and pressing into your hands.

2. For Cow, exhale and drop your stomach toward the floor, while looking straight ahead. Repeat back and forth slowly ten times. Meowing and mooing is optional.

Target body areas:

core, chest, spine, wrists, back, and shoulders.

Sports it benefits

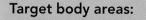

EAGLE FORWARD FOLD

(Garudasana Uttanasana)

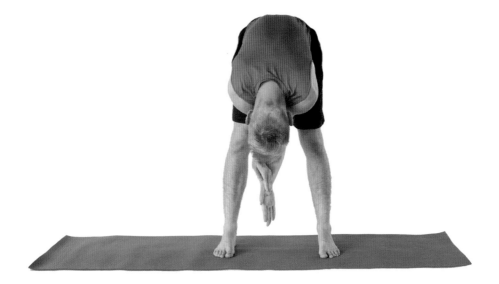

Once again, adding Eagle arms to a pose makes it a super pose, not to mention a huge release to your hamstrings.

1. From standing position, inhale and wrap your left arm under your right into Eagle arms.

2. Exhale and slowly dive down into Forward Fold, while placing your weight in the toes. Hold for five to ten deep breaths, and repeat with Eagle arms on the other side. It's a really cool feeling.

Target body areas:

calves, hamstrings, wrists, forearms, lower back, back, and shoulders.

Sports it benefits

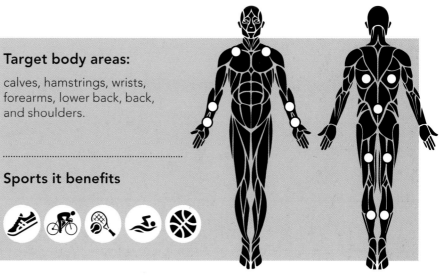

129

FIRELOG

(Dwapada Rajakapotasana)

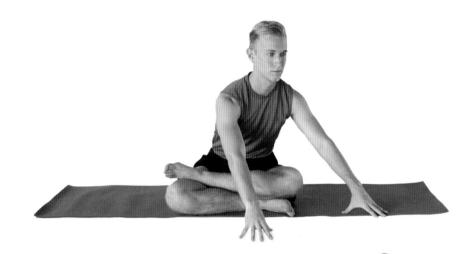

Throw some logs on the fire to really open up those hips.

1. From a cross-legged position, exhale and place your left ankle on your right thigh.

2. Inhale as you extend your arms overhead, and exhale as you lengthen off your left knee. Hold for five to ten deep breaths, and repeat on the other side.

Target body areas:

knees, gluteus, hips, and lower back.

Sports it benefits

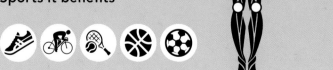

CATCHER'S SQUAT

(Nishadita Asana)

Here's how a Squat can really open up your hips.

1. From a standing position, exhale and squat down so your knees open to the sides.

2. Inhale and bring your palms together, and exhale as you press your tailbone toward the floor.

3. Inhale, lift your upper body, and use your elbows to open your hips farther. Hold for five to ten deep breaths, and slowly stand up.

Target body areas:

knees, quadriceps, hamstrings, gluteus, hips, and lower back.

Sports it benefits

KNEES IN
(Apanasana)

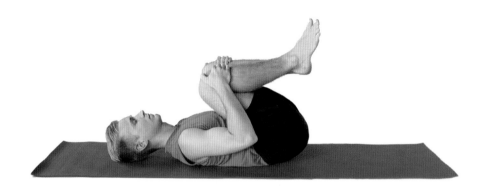

Give yourself a hug, and keep your lower back very happy. This stretch also calms and soothes the mind.

1. Lie on your back, and inhale as you draw your knees into your chest with your hands.

2. Exhale as you rock slowly to the side, and inhale as you return to the center. Rock side to side for five to ten deep breaths. Added bonus: Wiggle your fingers and toes.

Target body areas:

knees and lower back.

Sports it benefits

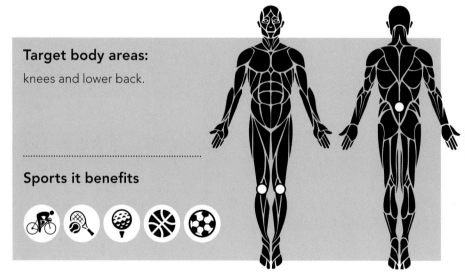

SUPINE BUTTERFLY/CORPSE
(Supta Baddha Konasana/Savasana)

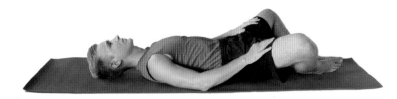

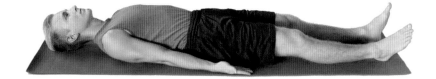

We've made it to the final two poses designed to take you right into the deepest sleep you've ever had. Corpse pose should be done for at least five minutes a day.

1. From Knees In position, inhale and bring the bottoms of your feet together. Exhale and drop them to the floor.

2. Place your hands on your inner thighs to help open the hips farther as you arch your back, relax your shoulders, and focus on five to ten deep breaths.

3. Exhale and slide your legs onto the floor into the beloved Corpse pose, the final pose of most yoga workouts.

4. Let your arms fall to the sides, relax your hips, and take five to ten deep breaths. After all the poses you've done, take some time to breathe, relax, and let your mind wander.

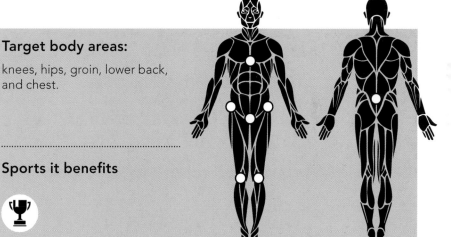

Target body areas:

knees, hips, groin, lower back, and chest.

Sports it benefits

133

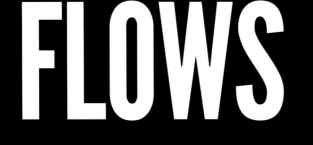

FLOWS

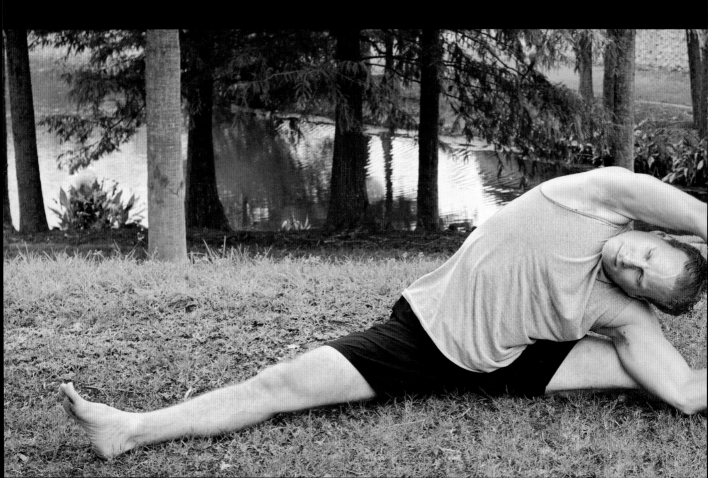

WARM-UP/ COOL-DOWN FLOWS

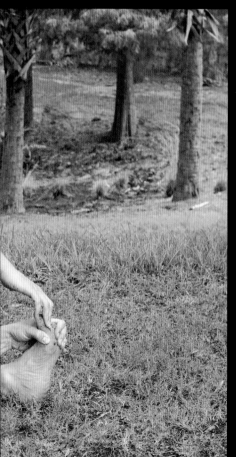

NOTE: As you practice these flows, I suggest you approach them in three ways:

1. As a beginner or someone wanting a deeper stretch, hold each pose for five to ten deep breaths (thirty to sixty seconds) to dig deep and emphasize a deep muscle burn and stretch. With this approach, the flows will be longer, but you'll be able to master the poses and move on to #2 and #3.

2. Hold each pose for only one or two breaths to raise your heart rate and create a more vigorous power yoga flow.

3. Vary the durations of each pose depending on how you're feeling. Make it your own!

These are the flows to get your blood flowing before your workout or gently wind down and release tension after a tough workout. Be sure to follow the sequence of the poses as given. You'll always need a little extra time to bridge the gap from your yoga workouts back into the real world and vice versa. As you hold each pose, let your breath take you deeper into each stretch. Your breath always defines the pose. Now, let's get loose!

BASIC STANDING WARM-UP FLOW

You're just getting started and need something gentle and patient with your feet on the ground. This is the flow for you.

1. Mountain (*page 17*)

2. Side Bend (both sides) (*page 18*)

3. Back Bend (*page 19*)

4. Forward Fold (*page 20*)

5. Flat Back (*page 21*)

6. Walking Forward Fold (*page 85*)

7. Back Bend (*page 19*)

8. Side Bend (both sides) (*page 18*)

(Repeat as desired.)

1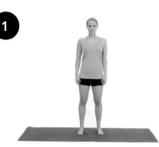

2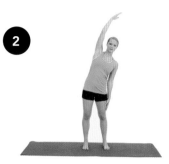

3

4

5

6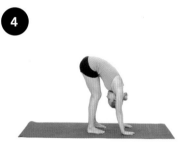

7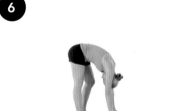

8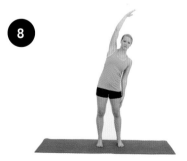

INTERMEDIATE WARM-UP FLOW

Let's add a couple more poses to sharpen your mind and get your blood flowing.

1. Mountain *(page 17)*
2. Tall Mountain *(page 29)*
3. Side Bend (both sides) *(page 18)*
4. Back Bend *(page 19)*
5. Chair *(page 27)*
6. Tall Mountain *(page 29)*
7. Walking Forward Fold *(page 85)*
8. Wide Legged Mudra *(page 79)*

(Repeat as desired.)

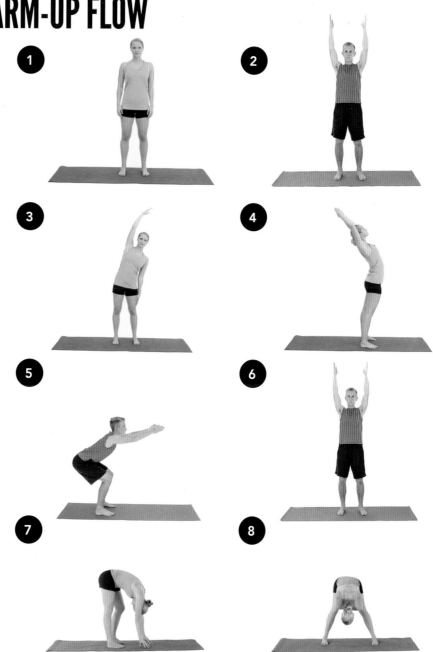

SWEATY AND READY WARM-UP FLOW

You're good to go for a spectacular workout after performing this flow. It will get your body heat revving and your sweat dripping.

1. Forward Fold (*page 20*)
2. Flat Back (*page 21*)
3. Walking Forward Fold (*page 85*)
4. Downward Facing Dog (*page 23*)
5. Classic Plank (*page 87*)
6. Upward Facing Dog (*page 25*)
7. Downward Facing Dog (*page 23*)
8. Forward Fold (*page 20*)

(Repeat as desired.)

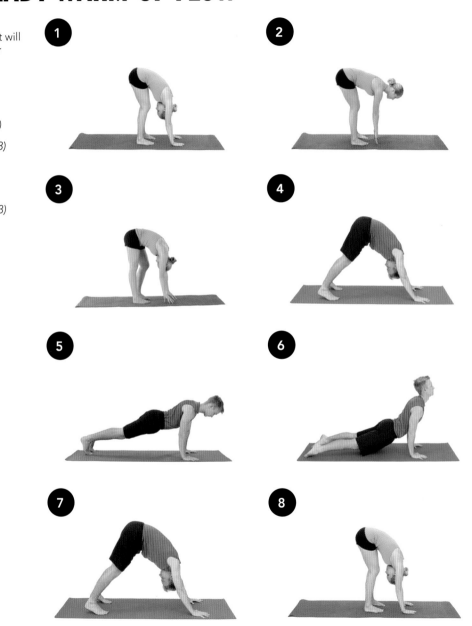

SUNRISE YOGA FLOW

Rise and shine! It's time for yoga and for beginning your day with a ton of energy! The sooner you get moving, the better your body will respond to all the challenges throughout the day.

1. Corpse (page 133)

2. Knees In (page 132)

3. Lying Spinal Twist (both sides) (page 125)

4. Supine Butterfly (page 133)

5. Spider (both legs) (page 123)

6. Happy Baby (page 124)

7. Knees In (page 132)

8. Low Lunge (both sides) (page 120)

(Repeat as desired.)

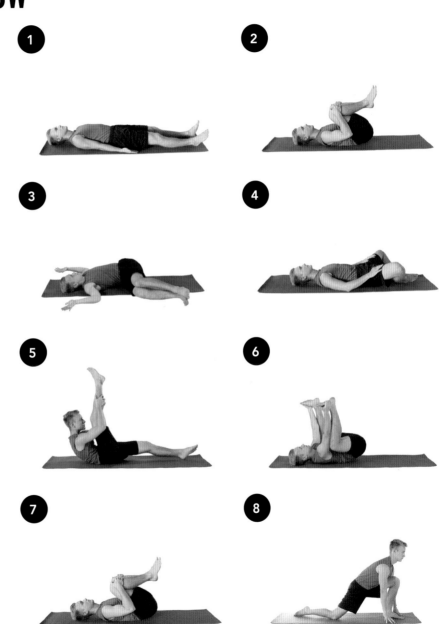

SUNSET YOGA FLOW

It's proven that doing yoga before bed will help you attain a deeper sleep with fewer distractions. You've trained hard all day and deserve to let go. Sweet dreams.

1. Mountain *(page 17)*

2. Side Bend (both sides) *(page 18)*

3. Forward Fold *(page 20)*

4. Downward Facing Dog *(page 23)*

5. Low Lunge (both sides) *(page 120)*

6. Child's Pose *(page 119)*

7. Thread the Needle (both sides) *(page 119)*

8. Cat *(page 128)*

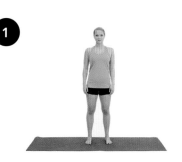

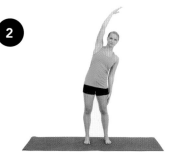

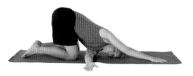

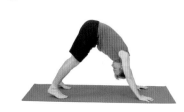

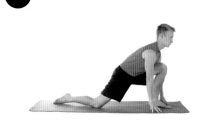

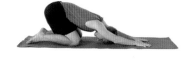

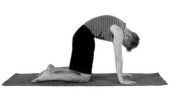

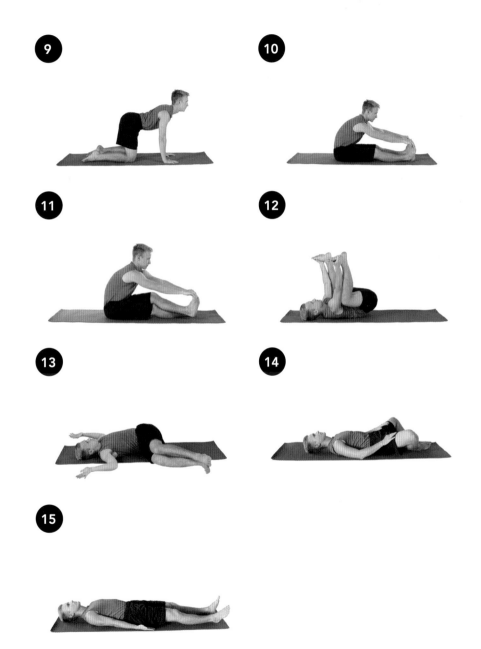

POST-WORKOUT FLOW

Pressed for time but really need to release those muscles? Here's a short flow to stretch your hamstrings, hip flexors, and lower back. Repeat this sequence on both sides.

1. Forward Fold *(page 20)*

2. Wide Legged Down Dog *(page 26)*

3. Downward Facing Dog *(page 23)*

4. Three Legged Dog *(page 24)*

5. Crescent Lunge *(page 74)*

6. Low Lunge *(page 120)*

7. Runner's Stretch *(page 127)*

8. Pigeon *(page 36)*

(Repeat steps 1–8 on the other side before continuing.)

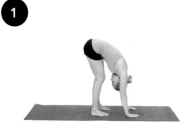

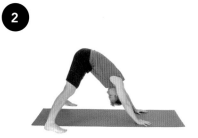

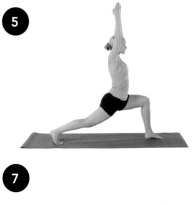

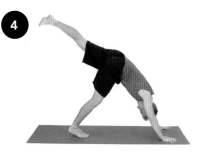

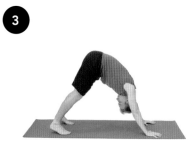

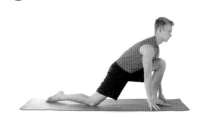

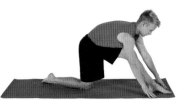

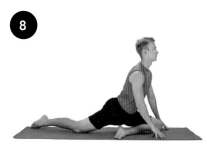

9. Child's Pose *(page 119)*
10. Thread the Needle (both sides) *(page 119)*
11. Straddle *(page 122)*
12. Folding Leaf *(page 121)*
13. Happy Baby *(page 124)*
14. Lying Spinal Twist (both sides) *(page 125)*

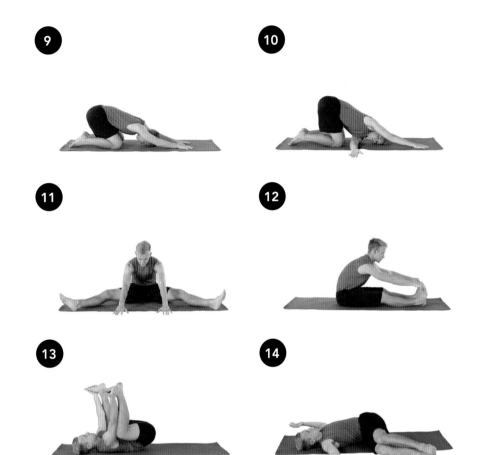

STANDING POST-WORKOUT FLOW

Get a massive total-body stretch for recovery, while keeping your feet planted firmly on the floor.

1. Mountain *(page 17)*
2. Back Bend *(page 19)*
3. Side Bend (both sides) *(page 18)*
4. Wide-Legged Mudra *(page 79)*
5. Wide-Legged Twist (both sides) *(page 117)*
6. Tall Mountain *(page 29)*
7. Forward Fold *(page 20)*
8. Walking Forward Fold *(page 85)*

(Repeat steps 1–8 on the other side.)

1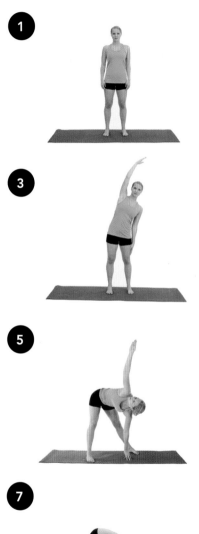

2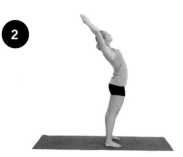

3

4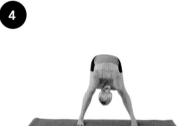

5

6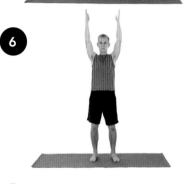

7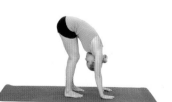

8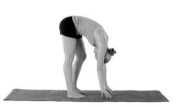

9. Downward Facing Dog *(page 23)*
10. Three Legged Dog *(page 24)*
11. Triangle *(page 71)*
12. Eagle Lunge *(page 75)*
13. Eagle Forward Fold *(page 129)*
14. Downward Facing Dog *(page 23)*
15. Wide Legged Down Dog *(page 26)*
16. Downward Facing Dog *(page 23)*

(Repeat steps 9–16 on the other side.)

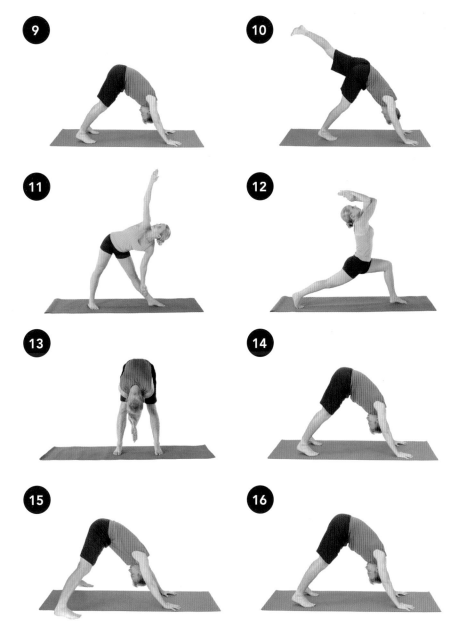

HIPS AND HAMSTRINGS STRETCH FLOW

Do this flow at the gym, on the go, or in front of the TV.

1. Tall Mountain *(page 29)*

2. Forward Fold *(page 20)*

3. Flat Back *(page 21)*

4. Walking Forward Fold *(page 85)*

5. Downward Facing Dog *(page 23)*

6. Cat *(page 128)*

7. Cow *(page 128)*

8. Thread the Needle (both sides) *(page 119)*

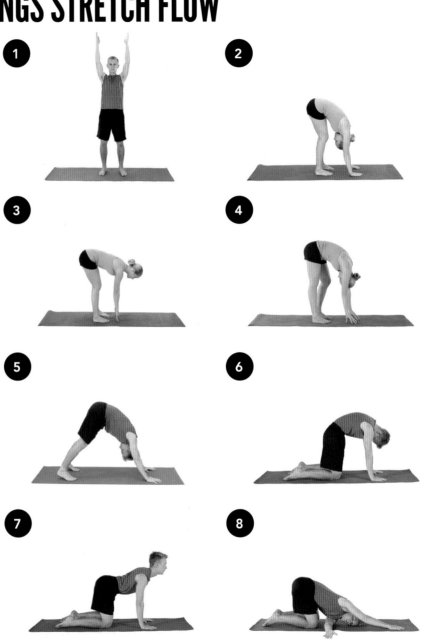

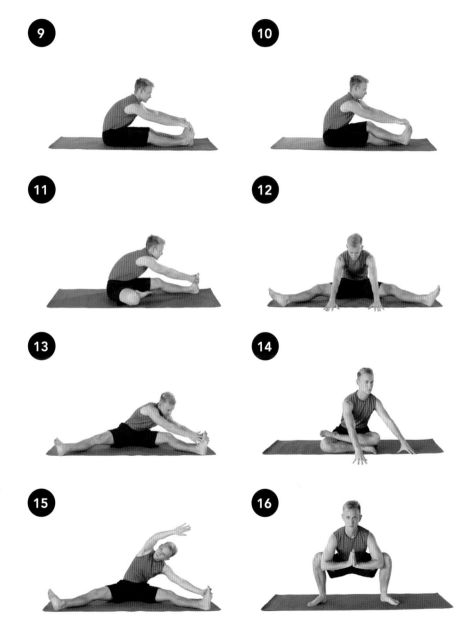

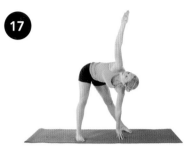
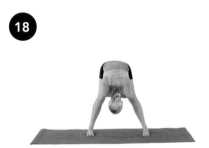

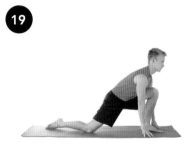
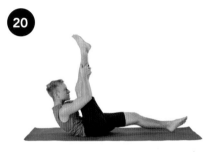

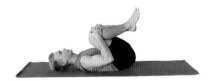

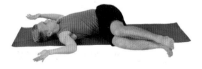
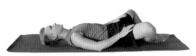

SEAN VIGUE'S PERSONAL YOGA STRETCH FLOW

Here's my go-to stretching routine when my body feels achy and tight. If I miss a day of stretching, my body will really give me hell for it. The more I stretch, the better I feel, and I recover much quicker to stay on my training schedule.

1. Mountain *(page 17)*
2. Walking Forward Fold *(page 85)*
3. Back Bend *(page 19)*
4. Downward Facing Dog *(page 23)*
5. Three Legged Dog *(page 24)*
6. Crescent Lunge *(page 74)*
7. Mudra Warrior *(page 62)*
8. Lunge Twist (both directions) *(page 84)*

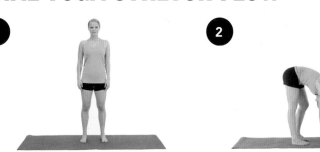

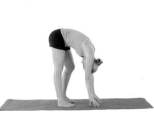

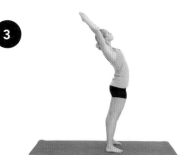

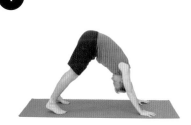

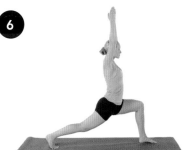

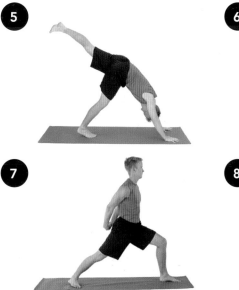

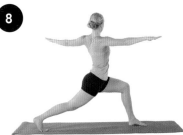

POWER YOGA FOR ATHLETES

9. Pigeon *(page 36)*

10. Walking Forward Fold *(page 85)*

11. Wide Legged Mudra *(page 79)*

12. Downward Facing Dog *(page 23)*

(Repeat steps 1–12 before continuing.)

13. Wide Legged Down Dog *(page 26)*

14. Pyramid (both sides) *(page 127)*

15. Catcher's Squat *(page 131)*

16. Straddle *(page 122)*

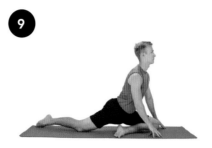

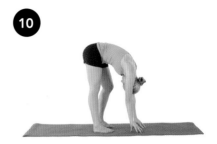

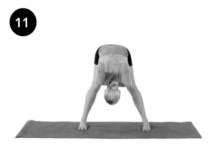

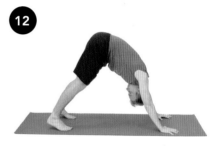

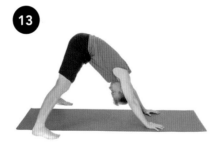

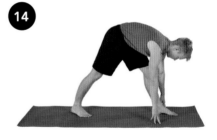

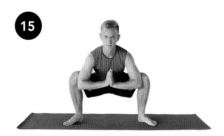

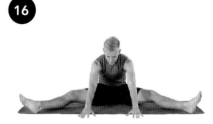

17. Straddle Twist (both sides) *(page 122)*

18. Side Bend Straddle (both sides) *(page 122)*

19. Spider (both legs) *(page 123)*

20. Happy Baby *(page 124)*

21. Lying Spinal Twist (both sides) *(page 125)*

22. Knees In *(page 132)*

23. Supine Butterfly *(page 133)*

24. Corpse (10 deep breaths) *(page 133)*

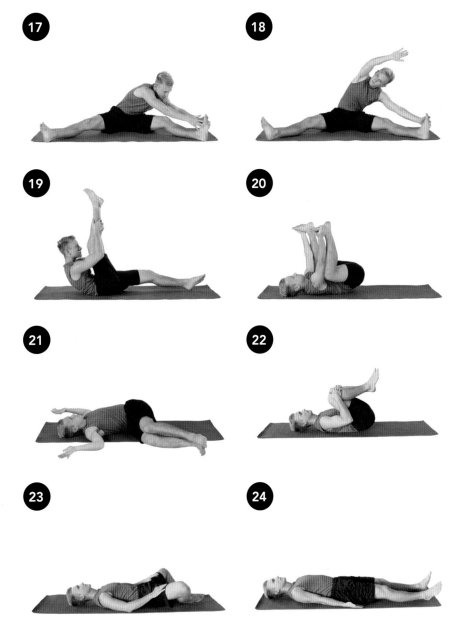

FULL BODY YOGA STRETCH FOR ENERGY AND STRENGTH

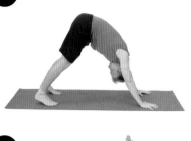

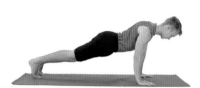

Sometimes I enjoy mixing my favorite core poses with deep stretching for a maximum post-workout strength and energy blast. The feeling is incredible! Let's begin in Downward Facing Dog...

1. Downward Facing Dog *(page 23)*
2. Classic Plank *(page 87)*
3. Side Plank (both sides) *(page 91)*
4. Camel *(page 28)*
5. Dolphin *(page 34)*
6. Camel *(page 28)*
7. Downward Facing Dog *(page 23)*
8. Forearm Plank *(page 88)*

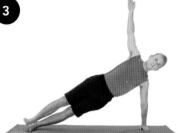

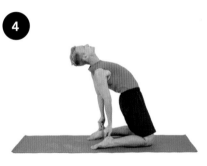

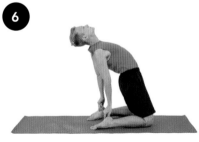

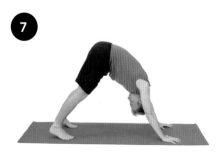

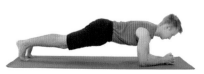

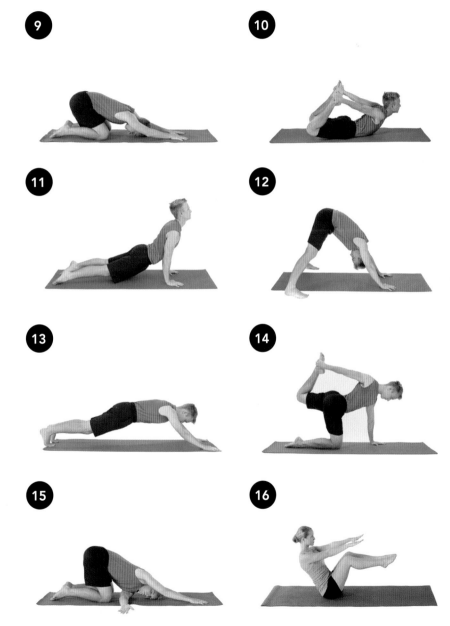

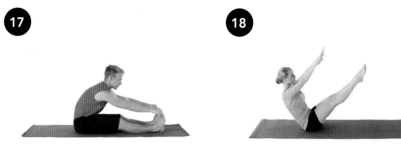

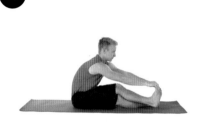

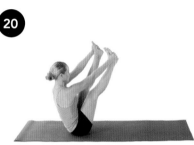

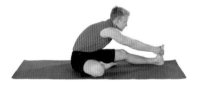

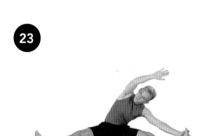

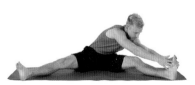

YOUR *POWER YOGA FOR ATHLETES* COMPLETE STRETCH FLOW

If you've got the time, I've got the flow to soothe and lengthen all of those spent muscles and sharpen your focus. As an athlete, you must renew every day to stay at the top of your game. These deep stretches will keep your body strong and ready for whatever challenges you face in your athletic endeavors.

1. Mountain *(page 17)*
2. Forward Fold *(page 20)*
3. Back Bend *(page 19)*
4. Downward Facing Dog *(page 23)*
5. Classic Plank *(page 87)*
6. Upward Facing Dog *(page 25)*
7. Downward Facing Dog *(page 23)*
8. Chair Twist (both sides) *(page 78)*

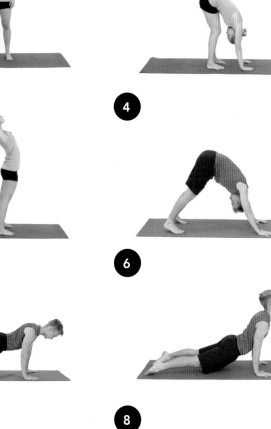

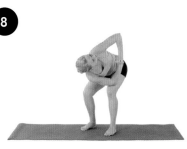

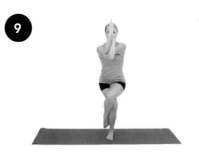

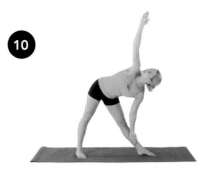

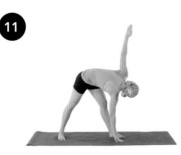

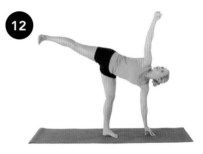

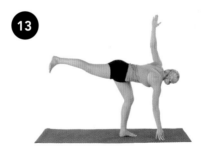

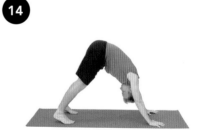

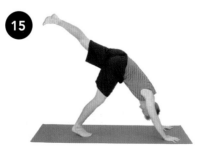

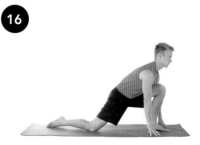

17. Crescent Lunge *(page 74)*

18. Eagle Lunge *(page 75)*

19. Pigeon *(page 36)*

20. Pyramid *(page 127)*

(Repeat steps 9–20 on the other side before continuing.)

21. Straddle *(page 122)*

22. Straddle Twist (both sides) *(page 122)*

23. Side Bend Straddle (both sides) *(page 122)*

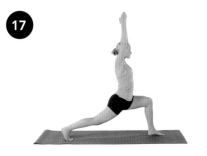
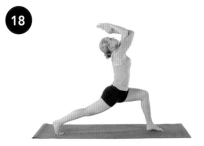
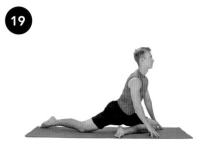
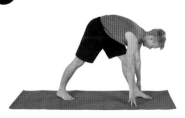
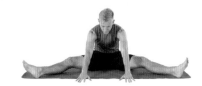
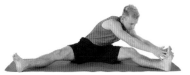
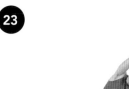
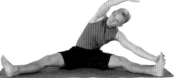

CHAPTER 10
POWER FLOWS

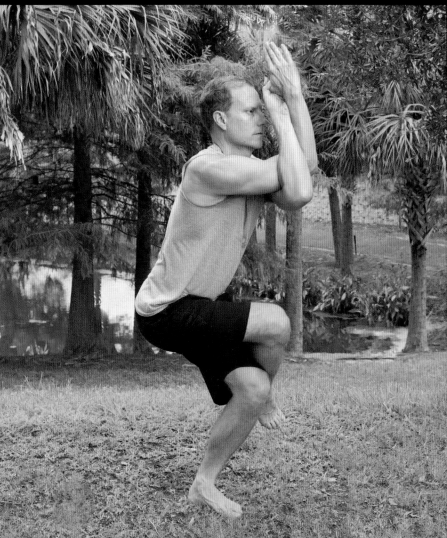

Crunched for time but need a killer workout? These powerful flows will have you sweating and stretching in no time at all. And they fit into even the busiest schedule. Try them before or after your normal workouts for optimum results, and feel free to repeat them as your time allows. I recommend holding each pose for one or two deep breaths, or holding longer if you want to dig deeper into a specific posture, and breathing into the transition from pose to pose. Repeat full sequences as many times as you like, and listen to your body. I enjoy holding the poses that are tougher for me for at least five breaths to make sure I fix my weaknesses and imbalances.

POWER VINYASA FLOW

This is the basic flow of power yoga, so take it slow, and allow every muscle to take part.

1. Mountain (*page 17*)
2. Forward Fold (*page 20*)
3. Flat Back (*page 21*)
4. Forward Fold (*page 20*)
5. Downward Facing Dog (*page 23*)
6. Classic Plank (*page 87*)
7. Hover Plank (*page 94*)
8. Upward Facing Dog (*page 25*)
9. Downward Facing Dog (*page 23*)
10. Mountain (*page 17*)

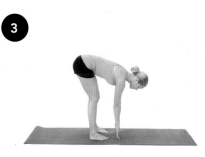

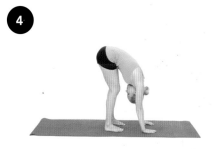

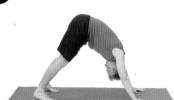

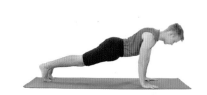

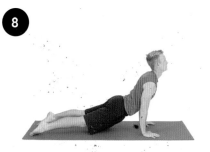

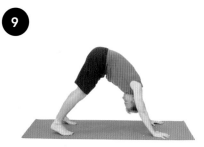

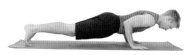

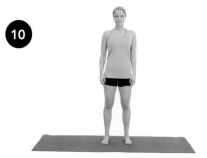

LUNGE VINYASA FLOW

Let's add a Lunge to the flow for increased balance and focus.

1. Downward Facing Dog *(page 23)*
2. Three Legged Dog *(page 24)*
3. Crescent Lunge *(page 74)*
4. Classic Plank *(page 87)*
5. Hover Plank *(page 94)*
6. Upward Facing Dog *(page 25)*
7. Downward Facing Dog *(page 23)*

(Repeat this sequence on the other side.)

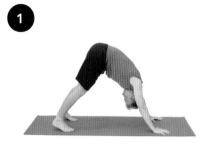

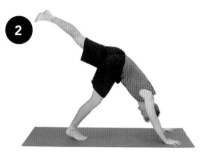

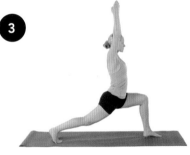

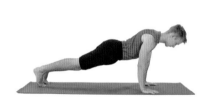

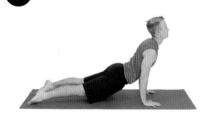

CORE POWER VINYASA FLOW

Build your powerful core, while stretching every muscle.

1. Mountain *(page 17)*
2. Forward Fold *(page 20)*
3. Downward Facing Dog *(page 23)*
4. Three Legged Dog *(page 24)*
5. Leg Lift Plank *(page 98)*
6. Hover Plank *(page 94)*
7. Upward Facing Dog *(page 25)*
8. Downward Facing Dog *(page 23)*

(Repeat this sequence on the other side.)

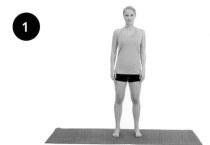

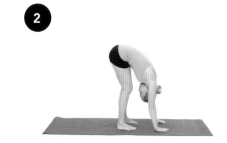

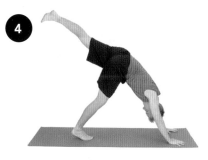

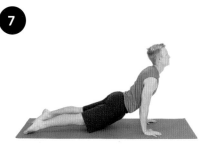

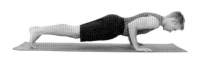

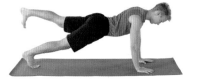

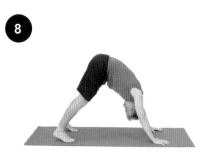

GEOMETRIC TRIANGLE FLOW

Pack on leg, gluteus, and core power with these posture-fixing Triangle variations.

1. Mountain *(page 17)*

2. Back Bend *(page 19)*

3. Chair *(page 27)*

4. Triangle *(page 71)*

5. Extreme Triangle *(page 72)*

6. Reverse Triangle *(page 73)*

7. Triangle *(page 71)*

8. *Mountain (page 17)*

(Repeat this sequence on the other side.)

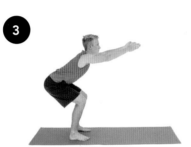
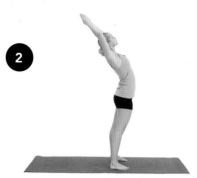
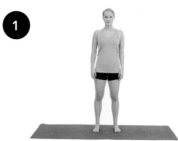
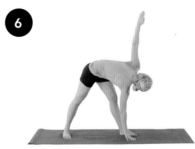
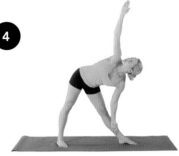
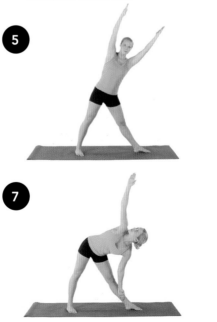
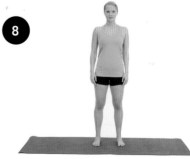

GLUTEUS BURNING CHAIR AND EAGLE FLOW

If you're looking for more gluteus and leg power, this is your flow.

1. Mountain *(page 17)*
2. Chair *(page 27)*
3. Chair Twist (both sides) *(page 78)*
4. Eagle (both sides) *(page 46)*
5. One-Legged Chair (both sides) *(page 47)*
6. Catcher's Squat *(page 131)*
7. Forward Fold *(page 20)*
8. Back Bend *(page 19)*

(Repeat as desired.)

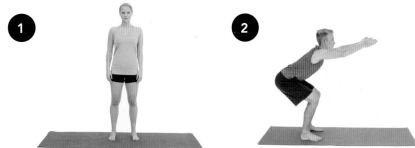

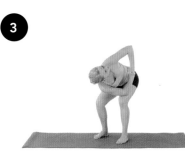

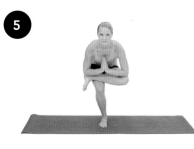

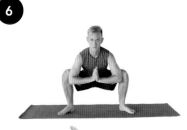

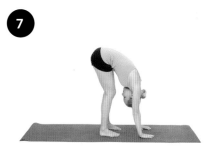

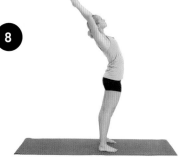

SEVERE TRIANGLE BALANCING FLOW

Challenge and fire up your muscles with the introduction of Half Moon poses to your training.

1. Mountain *(page 17)*

2. Triangle *(page 71)*

3. Extreme Triangle *(page 72)*

4. Half Moon (or Half Moon Balance) *(page 80)*

5. Revolving Half Moon (or Revolving Half Moon Balance) *(page 81)*

6. Standing Splits *(page 82)*

7. Half Moon (or Half Moon Balance) *(page 80)*

8. Triangle *(page 71)*

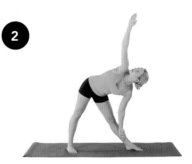

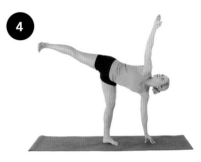

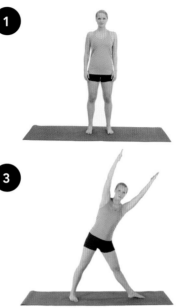

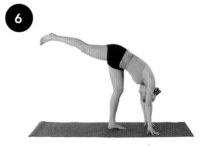

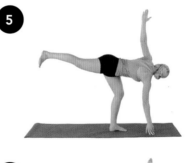

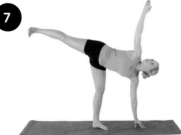

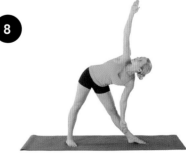

9. Tree *(page 39)*

10. Extended Tree *(page 40)*

11. Half Russian *(page 44)*

12. Standing Twist *(page 45)*

13. Triangle *(page 71)*

14. Mountain *(page 17)*

(Repeat this sequence on the other side.)

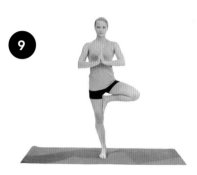

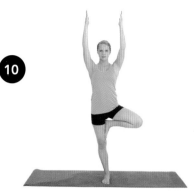

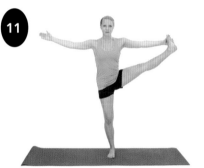

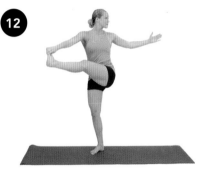

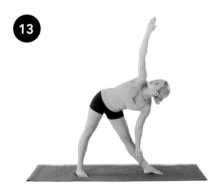

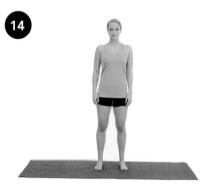

POWER PLANK FLOW

It's time to discover why Planks need to be every athlete's soul mate. You may also do the planks on your forearms.

1. Mountain (*page 17*)

2. Back Bend (*page 19*)

3. Forward Fold (*page 20*)

4. Downward Facing Dog (*page 23*)

5. Classic Plank (*page 87*)

6. Leg Lift Plank (both sides) (*page 98*)

7. Frozen Spiderman Plank (both sides) (*page 96*)

8. Reverse Plank (*page 89*)

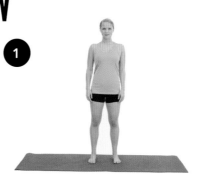
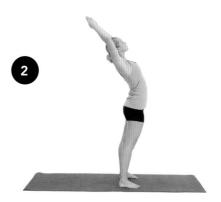
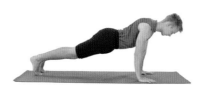
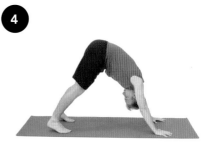
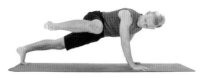
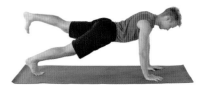
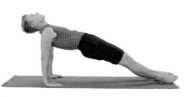

9. Popeye Plank *(page 99)*

10. Popeye Tap Plank (both sides) *(page 100)*

11. Bow *(page 33)*

12. Superman *(page 115)*

13. Classic Plank *(page 87)*

14. Hover Plank (to failure) *(page 94)*

15. Upward Facing Dog *(page 25)*

16. Child's Pose *(page 119)*

(Repeat as desired.)

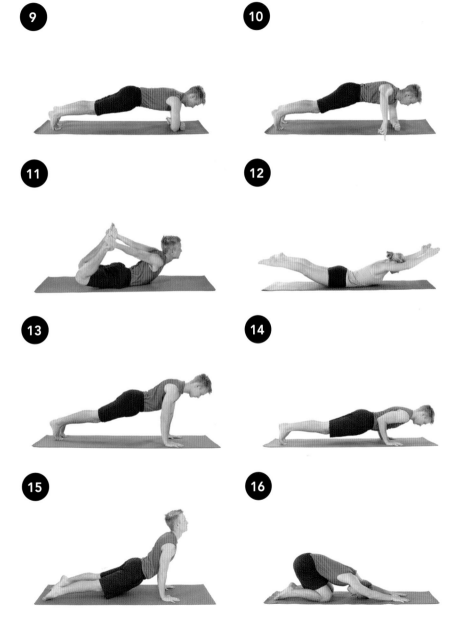

BALANCE AND ENERGY FLOW

Ratchet it up, and unleash your energy, core strength, and overall balance with this sweaty flow.

1. Mountain *(page 17)*
2. Tree (both sides) *(page 39)*
3. Dancer (both sides) *(page 43)*
4. Forward Fold *(page 20)*
5. Wide-Legged Mudra *(page 79)*
6. Chair *(page 27)*
7. Chair Twist (both sides) *(page 78)*
8. Warrior 3 (both sides) *(page 57)*

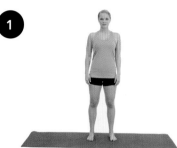

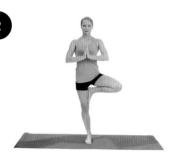

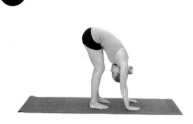

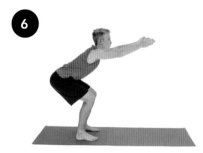

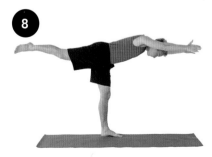

9. Downward Facing Dog *(page 23)*

10. Classic Plank *(page 87)*

11. Upward Facing Dog *(page 25)*

12. Child's Pose *(page 119)*

13. Shoulder Bridge/Wheel *(page 116)*

14. Mountain *(page 17)*

15. Eagle (both sides) *(page 46)*

16. Head to Knee (both sides) *(page 42)*

(Repeat sequence as desired.)

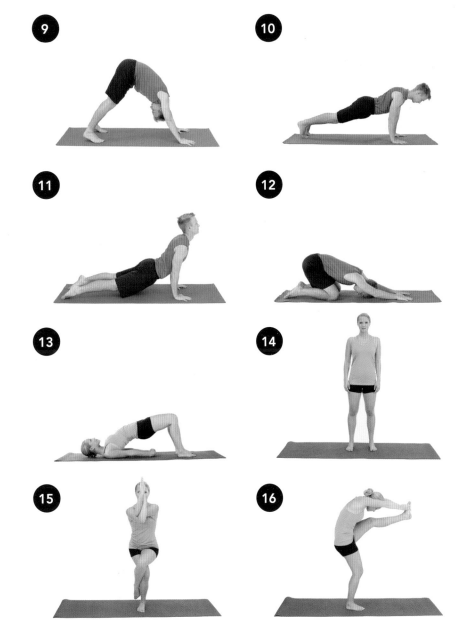

POWERFUL LEGS LUNGE AND WARRIOR FLOW

In a hurry, but need to experience and unleash your Lunge power? Here's an intense flow to bring instant balance, strength, and focus.

1. Mountain *(page 17)*
2. Forward Fold *(page 20)*
3. Downward Facing Dog *(page 23)*
4. Three Legged Dog *(page 24)*
5. Crescent Lunge *(page 74)*
6. Eagle Lunge *(page 75)*
7. Eagle Lunge Pointer *(page 76)*
8. Standing Splits *(page 82)*

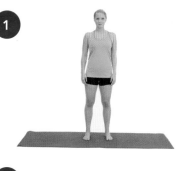

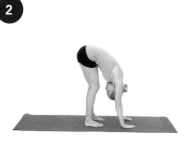

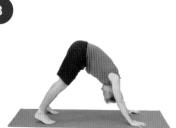

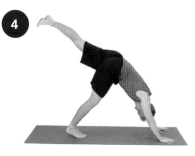

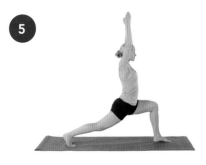

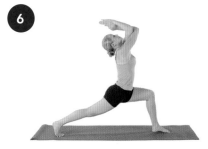

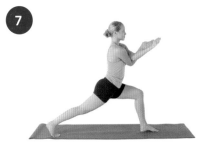

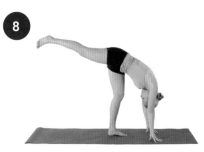

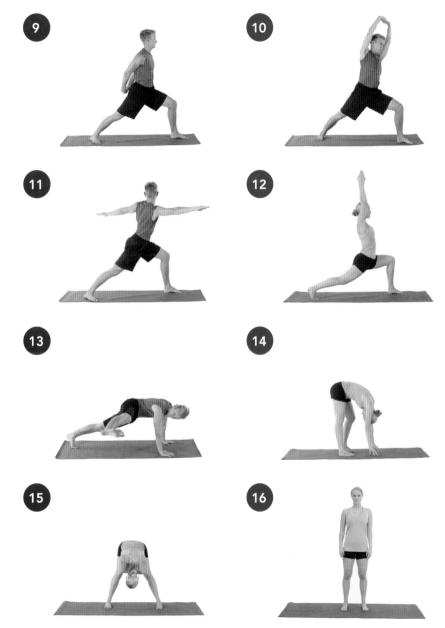

ULTIMATE WARRIOR AND BALANCE FLOW

This flow is all about unlimited endurance. Keep your control even as your legs begin to tremble.

1. Mountain *(page 17)*
2. Tree *(page 39)*
3. Star *(page 48)*
4. Shooting Star *(page 49)*
5. Dancer *(page 43)*

(Repeat steps 1–5 on the other side.)

6. Mountain *(page 17)*
7. Tall Mountain *(page 29)*
8. Side Bend (both sides) *(page 18)*

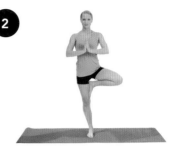

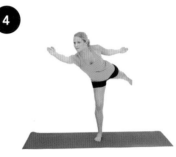

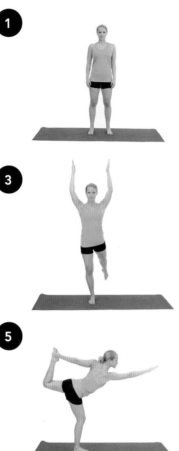

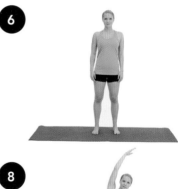

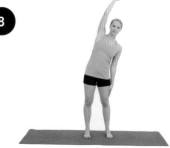

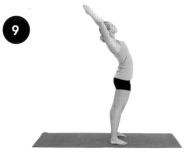

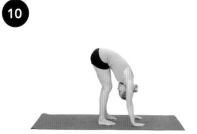

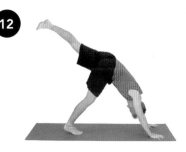

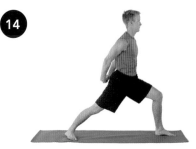

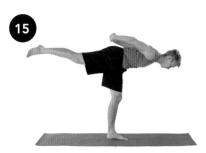

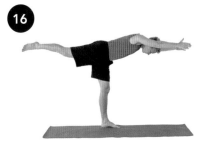

(Take a little breather before repeating 11–24 on the other side.)

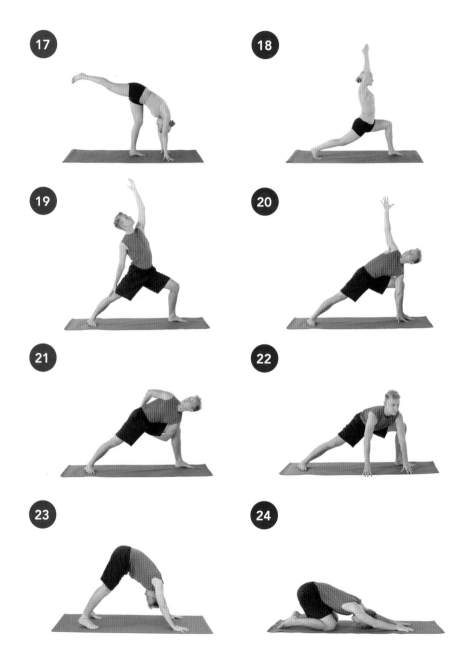

MUSCLE-SHREDDING POWER YOGA FLOW

This flow is all about shredding, sculpting, and lengthening your muscles. This is not for the faint of heart because there's an extra dose of those beautiful Plank variations. Now, take a deep breath (and many more), and prepare for glory!

1. Mountain (*page 17*)
2. Back Bend (*page 19*)
3. Chair (*page 27*)
4. Chair Twist (both sides) (*page 78*)
5. Forward Fold (*page 20*)
6. Dolphin (*page 34*)
7. Forearm Plank (*page 88*)
8. Walkout Plank (*page 90*)

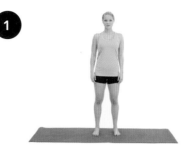
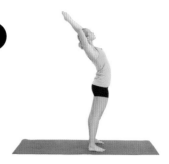
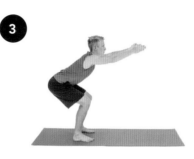
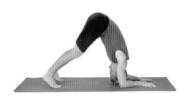

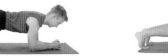
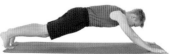

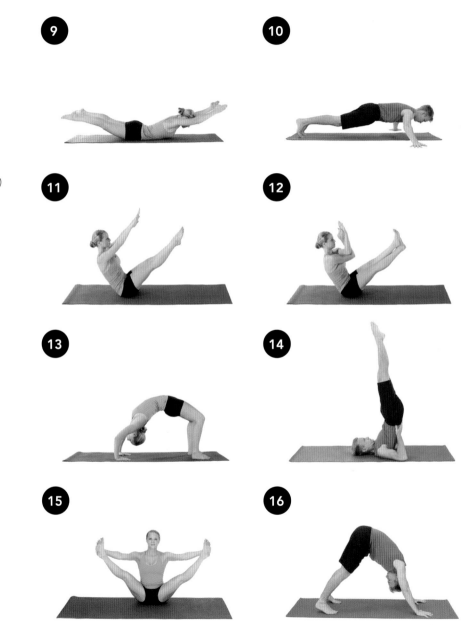

17. Hover Plank *(page 94)*
18. Upward Facing Dog *(page 25)*
19. Catcher's Squat *(page 131)*
20. Crow *(page 35)*
21. Hover Plank *(page 94)*
22. Upward Facing Dog *(page 25)*
23. Dolphin *(page 34)*
24. Cat Plank *(page 95)*

(Repeat as desired.)

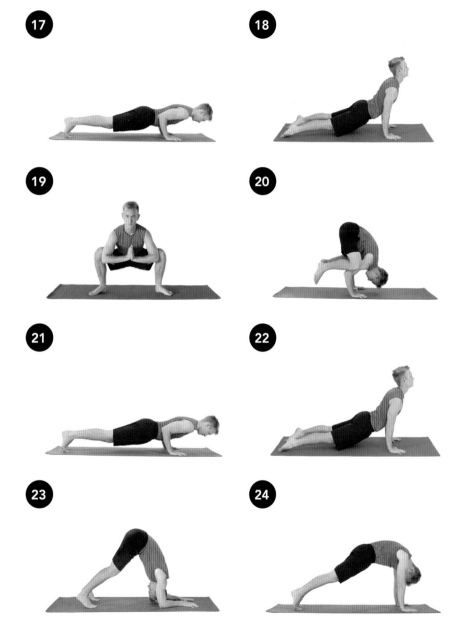

POWER YOGA HARD-CORE FLOW

What happens when you combine power yoga with core work? Extra speed, power, control, and mental focus. The final flow in this chapter is what you'll find me doing alone by the mirror at the gym. It's the ultimate in core strength and flexibility training. Every athlete who wants to be on the cutting edge must add this workout to their arsenal.

1. Downward Facing Dog *(page 23)*

2. Classic Plank *(page 87)*

3. Forearm Plank *(page 88)*

4. Bow *(page 33)*

5. Upward Facing Dog *(page 25)*

6. Classic Plank *(page 87)*

7. Nose to Knee Crunch (both sides) *(page 108)*

8. Child's Pose *(page 119)*

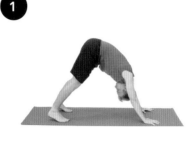

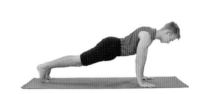

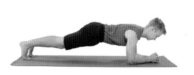

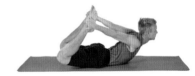

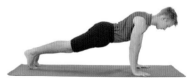

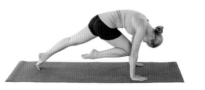

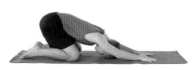

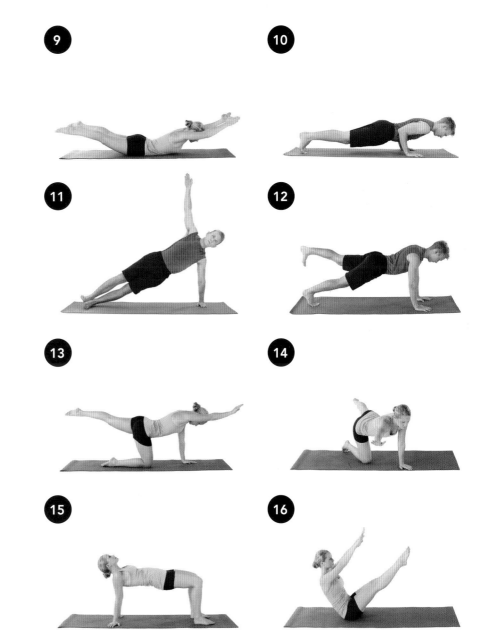

17. Wide-Legged Boat *(page 113)*

18. Wheel *(page 116)*

19. Full Boat *(page 110)*

20. Wheel *(page 116)*

21. Full Boat *(page 110)*

22. Knees In *(page 132)*

23. Extreme Boat *(page 114)*

24. Lying Spinal Twist (both sides) *(page 125)*

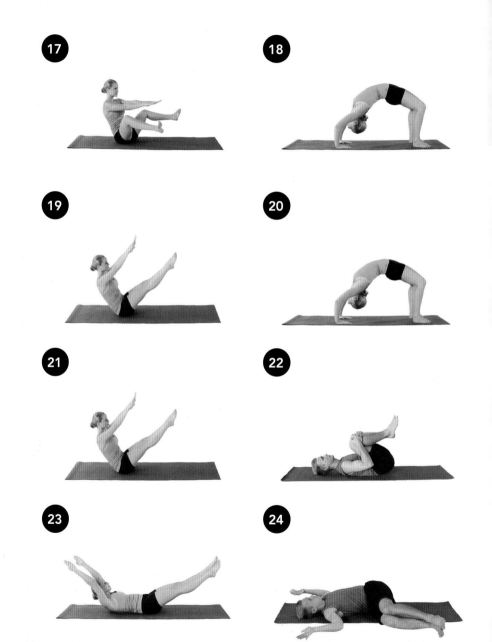

CHAPTER 11
ENDURANCE FLOWS

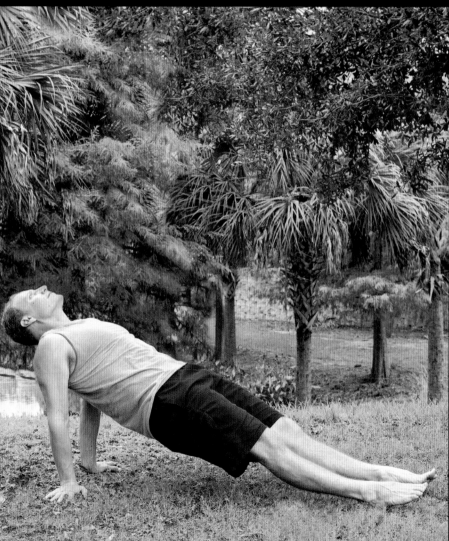

These are the two complete yoga workouts that make this book even more invaluable as your complete, portable power yoga training program! With these flows, we're going to work your body and mind to their full potential and build strong, long, lean muscles and incredible flexibility along the way. So, get ready to sweat those toxins out and experience the unrivaled effectiveness of power yoga and what it will do for your athletic performance. You may repeat each flow or combine several together—make the flows work for you, and modify them as needed. Hold every pose for one or two deep breaths, and breathe into the transitions for optimal results. Added bonus: Do these workouts with me (Sean) by visiting my YouTube channel at www.youtube.com/motleyfitness.

SEAN VIGUE'S PERSONAL POWER YOGA FLOW

This is my go-to flow when I need to shred some muscles, energize myself, build incredible power, and stretch my entire body. Repeat as many times as possible, and walk away feeling amazing! Caution: This may contain lots of planks, but that's only because I want you to be the best athlete you can be!

1. Walking Forward Fold *(page 85)*

2. Downward Facing Dog *(page 23)*

3. Classic Plank *(page 87)*

4. Walkout Plank *(page 90)*

5. Hover Plank *(page 94)*

6. Bow *(page 33)*

7. Superman *(page 115)*

8. Classic Plank *(page 87)*

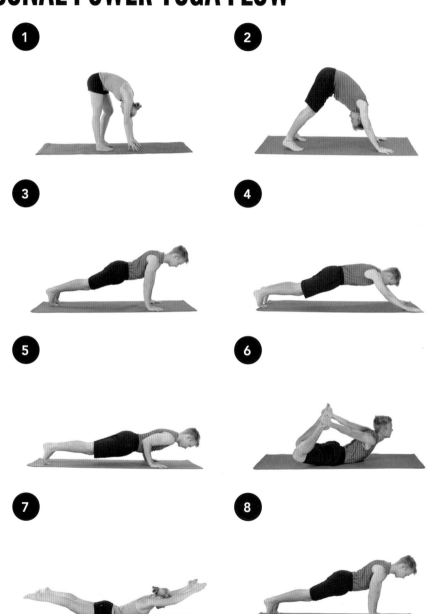

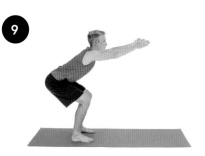

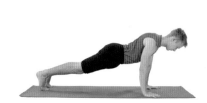

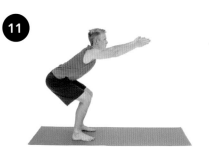

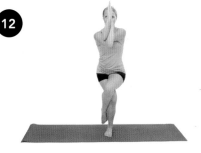

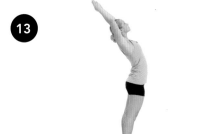

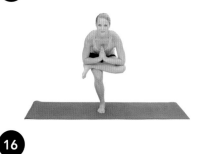

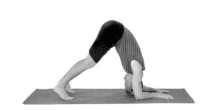

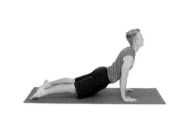
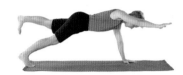
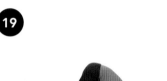
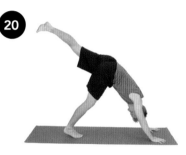
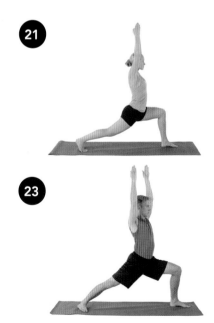
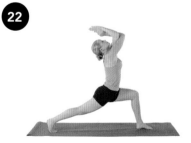
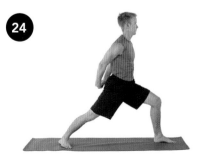

25. Mudra Warrior 3 *(page 63)*

26. Standing Splits *(page 82)*

(Repeat 19–26 on the other side before continuing.)

27. Full Boat *(page 110)*

28. Shoulder Bridge *(page 116)*

29. Extreme Boat *(page 114)*

30. Wheel *(page 116)*

31. Frozen Scissors (both sides) *(page 104)*

32. Extreme Boat (hold to failure, repeat as desired, and select a cool-down flow as the perfect finisher) *(page 114)*

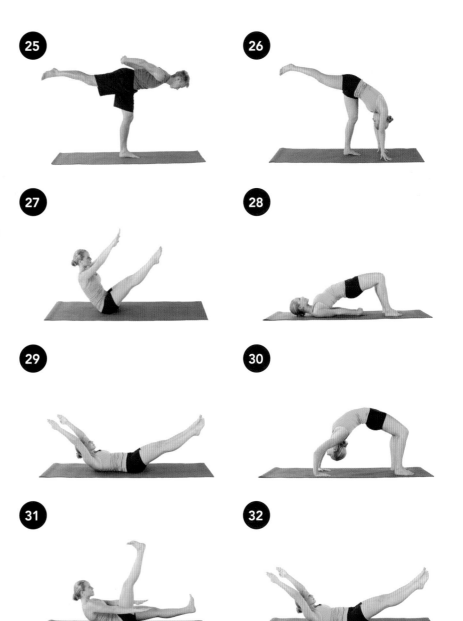

YOUR PERSONAL *POWER YOGA FOR ATHLETES* FLOW

This is the official flow of the book you're holding. You've trained hard and put your body through countless poses, and now it's time for your reward! This flow will have you sweating, digging deep, and, possibly, cursing. You're an athlete; be unstoppable. This is what we train for! Select a cool-down flow as the perfect finisher for this sequence.

1. Mountain *(page 17)*
2. Forward Fold *(page 20)*
3. Flat Back *(page 21)*
4. Classic Plank *(page 87)*
5. Hover Plank *(page 94)*
6. Upward Facing Dog *(page 25)*
7. Side Plank (both sides) *(page 91)*
8. Classic Plank *(page 87)*

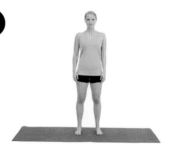
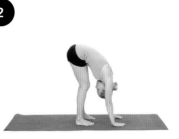
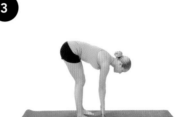
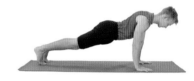
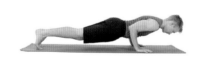
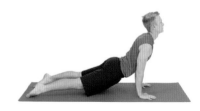
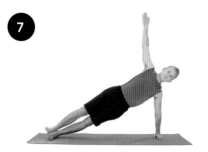

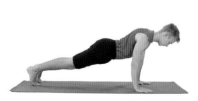

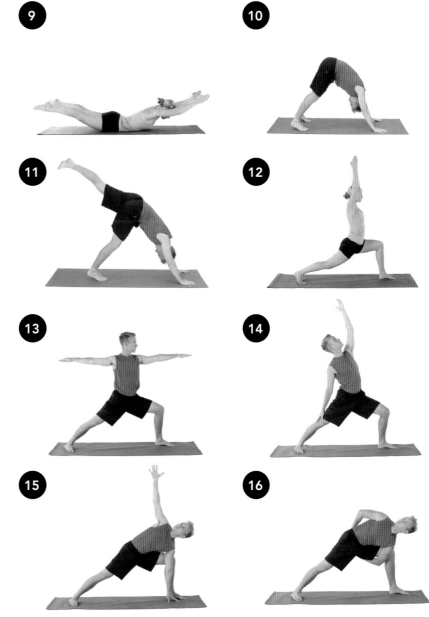

17. Reverse Warrior *(page 58)*

18. Half Moon Balance *(page 50)*

19. Revolving Half Moon Balance *(page 51)*

20. Standing Splits *(page 82)*

(Repeat steps 10–20 on the other side before continuing.)

21. Classic Plank *(page 87)*

22. Reverse Plank *(page 89)*

23. Extended Boat *(page 112)*

24. Crow *(page 35)*

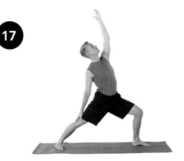

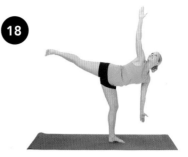

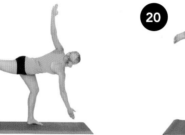

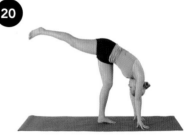

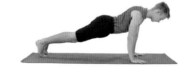

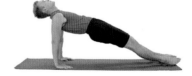

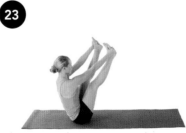

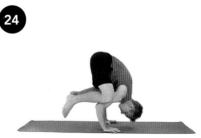

25. Balancing Bear *(page 52)*

26. Eagle Boat (both sides)
(page 111)

27. Balance the Cat (both sides)
(page 106)

28. Nose to Knee Crunch (both sides)
(page 108)

29. Frozen Scissors *(page 104)*
(both sides to failure)

30. Downward Facing Dog *(page 23)*

31. Walking Forward Fold *(page 85)*

32. Mountain *(page 17)*

(Repeat entire flow as many times as
desired.)

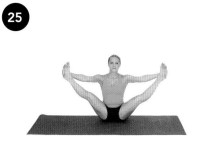

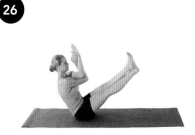

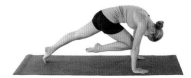

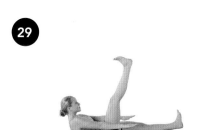

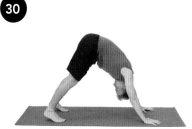

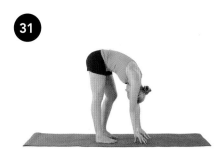

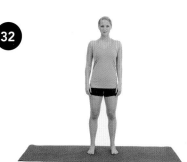

189

TRAINING LOG BY SPORT

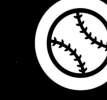

I created the Training Log for people looking to add yoga to their specific athletic training in the shortest amount of time. With well over 100 yoga poses contained in this book, it can be a little overwhelming to find the best poses for your training needs. To get started immediately, simply look up your sport or activity, and practice the recommended poses from the photos and descriptions in chapters 1 through 8. These are personally selected poses that will most benefit your specific training, but always keep in mind that every pose in this book will give you dynamic physical and mental benefits. The poses listed for each sport are arranged alphabetically for easy reference. For all the complete ready-made power yoga flows, check out chapters 9, 10, and 11. Add these poses into your current workout program, and hold each for five to ten deep breaths into your abdominals, while breathing in and out through your nose.

AMERICAN FOOTBALL/RUGBY

Since the Super Bowl XLVIII Champion Seattle Seahawks broke the news that their players practice yoga regularly, pro and amateur football clubs have been scrambling to get their players on a yoga program to see the same results. More and more gridiron warriors are flocking to yoga classes to improve their functional strength, balance, flexibility, power, breathing efficiency, speed, and focus, not to mention making them more resistant to injury and providing longevity in one of the most physically brutal sports in history. You just can't beat yoga's efficient combination of strength, flexibility, and focus, and it's giving football and rugby players around the world longer careers.

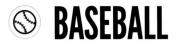

BASEBALL

Baseball and cricket demand fast reflexes, precise hand-eye coordination, tremendous speed after long periods of being inactive, and core strength to propel the ball between outfielders or knock it out of the park. Shortstops need to be agile and quick, pitchers need strong and flexible shoulders and core, catchers need balance and strong legs, hitters need a powerful core and flexible hips, and first basemen must have the flexibility to do the splits. Power yoga will keep your body strong, supple, and ready for all these demands and more. Here are the poses that are going to elevate and elongate your time on the field.

Awkward Airplane (page 107)	Lying Spinal Twist (page 125)
Back Bend (page 19)	Plow (page 31)
Balance the Cat (page 106)	Reach for the Sky (page 103)
Camel (page 28)	Reverse Triangle (page 73)
Cat/Cow (page 128)	Revolving Half Moon Balance (page 51)
Catcher's Squat (of course!) (page 131)	Runner's Stretch/Pyramid (page 127)
Chair (page 27)	Shoulder Stand (page 30)
Chair Twist (page 78)	Side Angle Warrior (page 59)
Child's Pose/Thread the Needle (page 119)	Side Bend (page 18)
Crow (page 35)	Spider (page 123)
Dolphin (page 34)	Spiderman Warrior (page 69)
Downward Facing Dog (page 23)	Standing Splits (page 82)
Flat Back (page 21)	Standing Twist (page 45)
Forward Fold (page 20)	Tree (page 39)
Frozen Scissors (page 104)	Triangle (page 71)
Full Boat (page 110)	Upward Facing Dog (page 25)
Gate (page 32)	Walking Forward Fold (page 85)
Half Boat (page 109)	Warrior 1 (page 55)
Half Moon Balance (page 50)	Warrior 3 (page 57)
Happy Baby (page 124)	Warrior Twist (page 68)
Hurdle (page 126)	Wide-Crescent Lunge (page 83)
Low Lunge/Splits (page 120)	Wide Legged Twist (page 117)
Lunge Twist (page 84)	

⚛ BASKETBALL

Here's a sport that's almost all running and jumping, causing tight hamstrings, lower back tension, shortened IT bands, and a sore gluteus, and has a high frequency of ankle sprains. Many top professional players have started utilizing yoga to stay flexible, build the muscles around their ankles, and give them added endurance to keep them running up and down the court smoothly. It's no wonder so many pro and college players are realizing the enormous edge these yoga poses will give you on the court.

Back Bend (page 19)	Pigeon (page 36)
Bow (page 33)	Plow (page 31)
Catcher's Squat (page 131)	Reverse Triangle (page 73)
Chair (page 27)	Reverse Warrior (page 58)
Dancer (page 43)	Revolving Half Moon (page 81)
Eagle Forward Fold (page 111)	Shoulder Bridge/Wheel (page 116)
Firelog (page 130)	Shoulder Stand (page 30)
Forward Fold (page 20)	Side Bend (page 18)
Full Boat (page 110)	Side Bend Warrior (page 67)
Half Moon (page 80)	Standing Half Moon (page 77)
Half Russian (page 44)	Standing Splits (page 82)
Handstand (page 53)	Straddle/Straddle Twist/Side Bend Straddle (page 122)
Happy Baby (page 124)	Tree (page 39)
Head to Knee (page 42)	Triangle (page 71)
Knees In (page 132)	Upward Facing Dog (page 25)
Low Lunge/Splits (page 120)	Warrior Wrap (page 61)
Lunge Twist (page 84)	Wide-Legged Twist (page 117)
Nose to Knee Crunch (page 108)	Willow (page 41)
One-Legged Chair (page 47)	

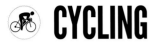

CYCLING

One of the best exercises on the planet is biking! Cyclists have strong, ripped legs, tons of endurance, acute mental focus, and super-revved-up metabolisms. With all of these powerful benefits, just imagine what more you could do with yoga. Well, you don't have to imagine anymore—yoga will give your cycling performance an incredible boost that will blow away your rivals!

The core strength and flexibility training of these yoga poses will give you the powerful speed, control, and focus you need for long, steady climbs or short bursts of sprints. You'll also stretch those tight hips and knees to keep you in the saddle for a long time. Let these poses elongate your love of biking.

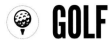

GOLF

I have been fortunate enough to train many professional and soon-to-be-professional golfers. The smart ones wandered into my classes because they needed a full-body fix to keep them on the links at 100 percent. Let's get right to the reason that golfers must do yoga: It will help your backswing, build and strengthen your core muscles, help you to hit longer drives, improve and fix your posture and lower your score. How? These poses will build strength and mobility in your hips, legs, and core, while generating more swing power from the ground up through your shoulders, arms, and, finally, into the club. Also, the deep, focused breathing relaxes your body, pumps oxygen into your muscles, and fixes the tension in your swings.

Cat/Cow (page 128)	Lying Spinal Twist (page 125)
Catcher's Squat (page 131)	Pigeon (page 36)
Child's Pose/Thread the Needle (page 119)	Reach for the Sky (page 103)
Crescent Lunge (page 74)	Reverse Warrior (page 58)
Dolphin (page 34)	Shoulder Bridge/Wheel (page 116)
Downward Facing Dog (page 23)	Side Angle Warrior (page 59)
Eagle (page 46)	Side Bend (page 18)
Eagle Boat (page 111)	Spider (page 123)
Eagle Forward Fold (page 129)	Standing Twist (page 45)
Eagle Lunge (page 75)	Star (page 48)
Eagle Warrior (page 64)	Supine Butterfly/Corpse (page 133)
Extended Boat (page 112)	Three Legged Dog (page 24)
Flat Back (page 21)	Tree (page 39)
Folding Leaf/Cross-Legged Folding Leaf (page 121)	Upward Facing Dog (page 25)
Forward Fold (page 20)	Walking Forward Fold (page 85)
Gate (page 32)	Warrior 1 (page 55)
Half Boat (page 109)	Warrior Twist (page 68)
Head to Knee (page 42)	Wide-Legged Mudra (page 79)
Hurdle (page 126)	Wide-Legged Twist (page 117)
Knees In (page 132)	

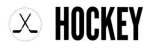

HOCKEY

I played hockey for 10 years, and I can tell you it's one of the most exciting yet grueling sports. It takes tremendous cardio capabilities combined with total control of your body as you fly down the ice, move through attackers, and dive for the puck. Hockey players also find it difficult to get proper recovery time with their heavy playing schedule and suffer from nagging injuries as a result of excessive exercise. Enter yoga. These poses will loosen and stretch your entire body, while keeping your core, legs, gluteus, and hips strong and resilient to injury. You'll also get extra power to slam your opponents mercilessly into the boards—if that's your thing.

Balance the Cat (page 106)	Mudra Warrior (page 62)
Camel (page 28)	Mudra Warrior 3 (page 63)
Chair (page 27)	One-Legged Chair (page 47)
Chair Twist (page 78)	Reverse Warrior (page 58)
Child's Pose/Thread the Needle (page 119)	Runner's Stretch/Pyramid (page 127)
Crab (page 105)	Shooting Star (page 49)
Crescent Lunge (page 74)	Side Bend (page 18)
Crow (page 35)	Spider (page 123)
Dancer (page 43)	Standing Half Moon (page 77)
Dolphin (page 34)	Superman (page 115)
Downward Facing Dog (page 23)	Supine Butterfly/Corpse (page 133)
Eagle (page 46)	Tiger (page 37)
Extreme Boat (page 114)	Upward Facing Dog (page 25)
Extreme Triangle (page 72)	Warrior 1 (page 55)
Flat Back (page 21)	Warrior 2 (page 56)
Folding Leaf/Cross-Legged Folding Leaf (page 121)	Warrior 3 (page 57)
Forward Fold (page 20)	Wide-Crescent Lunge (page 83)
Lunge Twist (page 84)	Wide-Legged Boat (page 113)
Lying Spinal Twist (page 125)	Wide-Legged Down Dog (page 26)

🏃 RUNNING/JOGGING

I have many clients in my classes and online who are runners, and their main complaint is always severe tightness: tight hamstrings, lower back, calves, hips, and shoulders. The tightness slows them down, drains their energy, and, in many cases, causes a lot of pain. I put together the yoga poses that will best help you loosen up, stand taller, and run farther with better posture. The breathing in yoga will also help you build endurance as you bring more oxygen into your body.

Balancing Bear (page 52)	Half Boat (page 109)
Bow (page 33)	Hurdle (page 126)
Camel (page 28)	Lying Spinal Twist (page 125)
Crescent Lunge (page 74)	Pigeon (page 36)
Dancer (page 43)	Reverse Warrior (page 58)
Downward Facing Dog (page 23)	Runner's Stretch/Pyramid (page 127)
Eagle Forward Fold (page 129)	Spider (page 123)
Eagle Lunge (page 75)	Straddle/Straddle Twist/Side Bend Straddle (page 122)
Firelog (page 130)	Superman (page 115)
Folding Leaf/Cross- Legged Folding Leaf (page 121)	Walking Forward Fold (page 85)
Frozen Scissors (page 104)	Wide-Legged Down Dog (page 26)
Full Boat (page 110)	

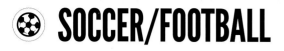 SOCCER/FOOTBALL

Here's the honest truth: soccer/football players can benefit from yoga because it causes improved flexibility, strength, and endurance. The tremendous agility required on the field will also be given a huge boost by adding yoga into your training, and your risk of injury will decrease. These poses will loosen and prepare your muscles for the strenuous exertion of a soccer game and the constant running, jumping, diving, kicking, sprinting, and even head butting that makes for a championship team. Let's go.

SWIMMING

Swimming is one of my favorite workouts because it's so easy on the joints and works my entire body in so many different ways. But too much time spent in the water with minimal resistance and lack of cross-training (doing other kinds of workouts) can cause body misalignments, tightness in the hips and shoulders, and lack of bone strength and density. My swimming clients are usually runners too, so I like to work with them on extending their muscles while building strength, balance, and flexibility. The longer and stronger you get on the mat, the faster you will be in the pool. Swimmers: Do these poses to tear it up in the pool!

Balance the Cat (page 106)	Lying Spinal Twist (page 125)
Child's Pose/Thread the Needle (page 119)	Plow (page 31)
Dolphin (page 34)	Proud Warrior (page 60)
Downward Facing Dog (page 23)	Revolving Half Moon Balance (page 51)
Eagle (page 46)	Shoulder Bridge/Wheel (page 116)
Eagle Lunge (page 75)	Straddle/Straddle Twist/Side Bend Straddle series (page 122)
Eagle Lunge Pointer (page 76)	Superman (page 115)
Eagle Warrior 3 (page 65)	Supine Butterfly/Corpse (page 133)
Extreme Boat (page 114)	Tree (page 39)
Full Boat (page 110)	Upward Facing Dog (page 25)
Half Moon Balance (page 50)	Warrior 1 (page 55)
Handstand (page 53)	Wide-Legged Down Dog (page 26)
Head to Knee (page 42)	Wide-Legged Mudra (page 79)

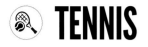

TENNIS

One of the toughest sports mentally is tennis. It's only you on the court, running back and forth, stopping and starting, sprinting, favoring one side of your body, chasing that ball, and trying to stay focused. I know because I played for many years but was unfortunate to not know about yoga. Yoga poses help players maintain muscular symmetry and improve their balance.

With all the physical demands of tennis, some players may develop tightness in their shoulders, arms, hips, and legs. These yoga poses are designed to improve core and leg strength, full-body flexibility, injury prevention, coordination, and stamina so you can zoom right through any tiebreaker and beyond.

INDEX

ACKNOWLEDGMENTS

Massive thanks to my beautiful wife, Jillian, for all her support during the exciting (and sometimes stressful) process of writing my first book. I'm so glad you came to my Pilates class back in 2007 and I wasted no time in asking you out! "I lives you."

To my parents, Bob and Beverly, and my sister Kim; you guys have always been my rock through the years (even during my twelve wild years in professional theater), and I love you very much. They all attend my classes when they visit and really love when I tell them to do Planks.

Big shout-out to my two best friends, SS and Peter. You guys have always pushed me to learn and grow not just my business but myself as a person, and I thank God for you every day. "You're gonna scare the hell out of those guys!"

To my photographer, Terri, and our two gorgeous models, Katelynn and Matt. You guys were so professional, fun, and patient as we made the bold choice to put more poses in this book than any other yoga book in history! Thank you for all your hard work.

To Bonnie Bauman for your invaluable help with proofreading and fixing my grammatical errors.

And finally to Jessica at Fair Winds Press, who found and offered me the amazing opportunity to write this book. You've been a real joy to work with, and thanks for putting up with my occasional bouts of being overwhelmed.

ABOUT THE AUTHOR

Sean is a yoga, Pilates, and spinning instructor who recently relocated to the mountains of Colorado from the swamps of central Florida. He has taught more than 5,000 group fitness classes, and his *Pilates for Men* DVD was named "Best Male Workout" by *Pilates Style* magazine. Sean is one of the most sought-after yoga and Pilates teachers in the world and has more than 1,000 workout videos on the market. You can follow him on his YouTube channel, youtube.com/motleyfitness, and website, SeanVigueFitness.com.

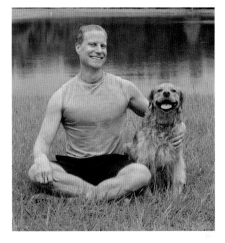

ABOUT THE PHOTOGRAPHER

Terri Zollinger, a lifestyle photographer for 8 years, loves to visually document life. Photography has always been an interest but became very prevalent in her life after having her children. One thing led to another and Terri Z Photography was created. Terri Z Photography has been growing strong ever since and captures first steps, milestones, life changing moments, and marketing images for her clients across the U.S. To date, she has worked with more than 400 clients and looks forward to the new adventures and possibilities they take her on with this journey. Terri Zollinger lives in Florida with her husband and two children. To see more of Terri's work, visit www.terrizphotography.com or email her at terri@terrizphotography.com

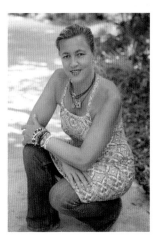

ALSO AVAILABLE

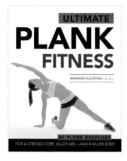

Ultimate Plank Fitness
978-1-59233-660-9

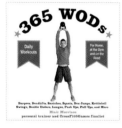

Core Fitness Solution
978-1-59233-640-1

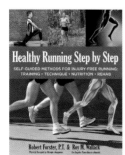

365 WODs
978-1-59233-637-1

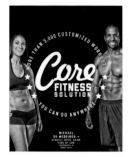

Healthy Running Step-by-Step
978-1-59233-605-0